The Skills of History Taking

For Medical Students and Practitioners

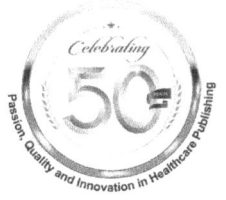

The Skills of History Taking

For Medical Students and Practitioners

(Based on AETCOM Module)

Third Edition

Rahul Tanwani MS MCh
Professor
Department of Surgery
Index Medical College, Hospital and Research Center
Indore, Madhya Pradesh, India

Foreword
DP Lokwani

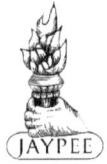

JAYPEE BROTHERS MEDICAL PUBLISHERS
The Health Sciences Publisher
New Delhi | London

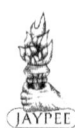 **Jaypee Brothers Medical Publishers (P) Ltd**

Headquarters
Jaypee Brothers Medical Publishers (P) Ltd
EMCA House, 23/23-B
Ansari Road, Daryaganj
New Delhi 110 002, India
Landline: +91-11-23272143, +91-11-23272703
+91-11-23282021, +91-11-23245672
Email: jaypee@jaypeebrothers.com

Corporate Office
Jaypee Brothers Medical Publishers (P) Ltd
4838/24, Ansari Road, Daryaganj
New Delhi 110 002, India
Phone: +91-11-43574357
Fax: +91-11-43574314
Email: jaypee@jaypeebrothers.com

Overseas Office
J.P. Medical Ltd
83 Victoria Street, London
SW1H 0HW (UK)
Phone: +44 20 3170 8910
Fax: +44 (0)20 3008 6180
Email: info@jpmedpub.com

Website: www.jaypeebrothers.com
Website: www.jaypeedigital.com

© 2021, Jaypee Brothers Medical Publishers

The views and opinions expressed in this book are solely those of the original contributor(s)/author(s) and do not necessarily represent those of editor(s) of the book.

All rights reserved. No part of this publication may be reproduced, stored or transmitted in any form or by any means, electronic, mechanical, photocopying, recording or otherwise, without the prior permission in writing of the publishers.

All brand names and product names used in this book are trade names, service marks, trademarks or registered trademarks of their respective owners. The publisher is not associated with any product or vendor mentioned in this book.

Medical knowledge and practice change constantly. This book is designed to provide accurate, authoritative information about the subject matter in question. However, readers are advised to check the most current information available on procedures included and check information from the manufacturer of each product to be administered, to verify the recommended dose, formula, method and duration of administration, adverse effects and contraindications. It is the responsibility of the practitioner to take all appropriate safety precautions. Neither the publisher nor the author(s)/editor(s) assume any liability for any injury and/or damage to persons or property arising from or related to use of material in this book.

This book is sold on the understanding that the publisher is not engaged in providing professional medical services. If such advice or services are required, the services of a competent medical professional should be sought.

Every effort has been made where necessary to contact holders of copyright to obtain permission to reproduce copyright material. If any have been inadvertently overlooked, the publisher will be pleased to make the necessary arrangements at the first opportunity. The **CD/DVD-ROM** (if any) provided in the sealed envelope with this book is complimentary and free of cost. **Not meant for sale.**

Inquiries for bulk sales may be solicited at: jaypee@jaypeebrothers.com

The Skills of History Taking for Medical Students and Practitioners

First Edition: **2014** (Published by Author)

Second Edition: **2016**

Third Edition : **2021**

ISBN 978-93-5465-087-1

Dedicated to
My family
and
My students

Foreword

An appropriate communication with his patients is a key to success of any practicing doctor. In clinical practice, most of the diagnoses can be made on the basis of history taking alone and excessive clinging to investigations may ruin and atrophy both clinical skills and practice.

It is my privilege to present a foreword for this excellent piece of work. The most desired and untouched subject of "history taking" has been addressed thoughtfully and meticulously. The proper way of history taking and its presentation, local terminologies, and the art of dealing with special cases are few of the impressive features. The tailor-made approach and Hindi questionnaire for interacting with patients are unique and will definitely help the students and the practitioners in the long way. Perhaps, the interaction of a student with a patient, before, during, and after history taking cannot be explained in a more precise and apt form.

The affection of this book to answer the most frequently faced problem, *how to ask*, is quite appreciable. In this regard, the concepts of Western world cannot be replicated for developing countries and the author has meticulously framed the methodology, which is quite suitable for our country.

I am sure that his hard work of all these years will be used by medical science in years to come. My best wishes for the success and meaningful utility of this book.

DP Lokwani
Former Vice-Chancellor
Madhya Pradesh Medical Science University
Jabalpur, Madhya Pradesh, India

Preface to the Third Edition

It gives me a feeling of immense pleasure and satisfaction to see the place of subject of *communication skills* in revised medical curriculum of our country. For so many years, this subject was taught and learnt in our institutes mostly at subconscious level. Our students were learning it mainly by observing the communication of their seniors and teachers with various types of patients. I am glad to find it as an essential part of our curriculum, as it will be of great help in the methodical teaching and assessment of this subject in future. I hope that all my work on this subject in previous years will prove itself of great value in future time.

I have tried my best to format this edition according to the structure and recommendations of novel AETCOM Module. Contents have been divided in various sections and chapters, for ease and better understanding of our students. Almost all recommendations and suggestions are supported by some real life examples, mainly to make them interesting and easy-to-understand by students and practicing doctors.

Every medical student will become a practicing doctor in future and every practicing doctor is constantly learning the art and skill of communication. I have tried my best to make this book valuable for both present and future life of our students. Also, a major significant focus has been made on the communication with different types of patients during clinical practice.

The contents of this book are based on my personal observations as well as on the ideas and suggestions generated by interacting with medical teachers, students, private practitioners, multiple patients, and their family members. As with the previous editions, I have tried my best to avoid any controversies in the text. Still, I apologize for any disagreement if it perhaps finds its way in.

As before, I welcome constructive criticism and suggestions from the readers for further improvement of the book.

I hope that this book will prove itself beneficial for the students in improving their communication skills with the patients both in their present as well as in future life.

Rahul Tanwani

Preface to the First Edition

Proper communication with patients is an art and every doctor keeps on learning and improving it throughout his life.

A patient visits a doctor with a diseased body, a pile of complaints, and a hope to get some remedy from him. By his skills of history taking and clinical examination, the doctor is able to diagnose what is troubling the patient and subsequently prescribes medications for the same. Improperly elicited history may mislead to a wrong diagnosis and hence, to an ineffective treatment. So, a proper communication with the patient is the key to success for medical therapy.

The art of history taking and physical examination is taught to a doctor, right from his student life in a medical college. Most of the literature available in our country has emphasized on examination of the patients and the practical aspects of history taking have been summarized only in initial few pages. Though this part has been extensively covered in foreign literature, but because of the significant difference in culture and lifestyle, it cannot be blindly replicated for students and patients of our country.

The skill of history taking is based on three basic questions: *What to ask?*, *Why to ask?*, and *How to ask?*. This book is pretty much intended to the most under covered of these three: "How to ask?", as the remaining two have been adequately covered by other available literatures, both by Indian and foreign authors.

Detailed description of proper history taking has been presented. To make it more interesting and perceptible for the students, almost every point is supported by suitable illustrations. In fact, these are the cases which I actually came across as a student, a doctor, and a teacher. Most of them are surgical cases, but this book should not be considered as a book of history taking of only surgical patients.

This book should be considered as a supplementary manual for general communication with patients and is based on my observation of the commonly encountered problems, by students, while communicating with different patients. These observations have been confirmed and augmented by interacting with consultants of various clinical departments, multiple students, patients, and their relatives.

Besides, there are many instructions which may not be very useful for students at present, but will play an important role in their future life, as a practicing doctor. Though this book primarily caters to the needs of medical students, it may be consulted by medical practitioners as well, to improve their interaction with patients in their clinical practice.

I acknowledge my gratitude to all my colleagues in the department who gave me unstinted support, especially to Dr GV Vivekanandan, Head, Department of Surgery, Index Medical College, Indore, Madhya Pradesh, India, for encouraging me throughout the process of writing this book. I also express my thanks to all the consultants from different clinical and paraclinical departments, for their valuable contributions.

I pay my sincere regard to Dr BR Parekh (Director Professor, Department of Pediatric Surgery, Shri Aurobindo Medical College and Postgraduate Institute, Indore) for blessing the contents of this textbook by his valuable suggestions and appropriate modifications. I acknowledge my gratitude to Dr DP Lokwani (Vice-Chancellor, Madhya Pradesh Medical Science University, Jabalpur, Madhya Pradesh) for blessing me by adding his foreword letter to the textbook.

I have tried my best to be cautious enough to avoid any controversies in the text. I however apologize for any, if they perhaps find their way in. I welcome comments concerning omissions and errors, reviews regarding content, and critical suggestions for further editions. They may be e-mailed to dr.tanwani.rahul@gmail.com.

I hope that this book will prove itself beneficial for the students in improving their communication skills with patients, as a medical student at present and as a practicing doctor in future.

Rahul Tanwani

Acknowledgments

I must begin with thanking my parents and teachers for making me what I am today.

I heartily thank all the readers of previous editions of this book, who encouraged me by their positive feedback and valuable suggestions.

I am thankful to Mr Suresh Singh Bhadoria, Chairman, Index Group of Institutions, Indore for giving me permission and desired help to work in the field of communication skills in his Institute. I express my sincere gratitude to the faculties of various departments of my college for their precious suggestions.

I pay my sincere regard to Late Dr BR Parekh (Former Professor and Head, Department of Pediatric Surgery, MGM Medical College, Indore) for his blessings and suggestions, right from the first edition of this book.

I am thankful to Dr DP Lokwani (Former Vice-Chancellor, MP Medical Science University, Jabalpur) for blessing my work with his foreword letter in its first edition and for constantly encouraging me to move ahead in this field.

I pay my regard to Dr (Mrs) Sukhwant Bose (Director Professor, Department of Physiology and Convener, MCI Regional Training Centre in Medical Education Technology, Shri Aurobindo Institute of Medical Science, Indore) for her blessings, guidance, and appreciations, right from the beginning of my academic career.

I heartily thank Shri Jitendar P Vij (Group Chairman), Mr Ankit Vij (Managing Director), Mr MS Mani (Group President), Dr Madhu Choudhary (Publishing Head-Education), Ms Pooja Bhandari (Production Head), Ms Sunita Katla (Executive Assistant to Group Chairman and Publishing Manager), Ms Samina Khan (Executive Assistant to Publishing Head-Education), Dr Aakanksha Shukla Sirohi (Development Editor), Mr Rajesh Sharma (Production Coordinator), Ms Seema Dogra (Cover Visualizer), Mr Vakil Khan (Proofreader), Mr Kulwant Singh (Typesetter), Mr Shravan Kumar (Graphic Designer) and their team members of M/s Jaypee Brothers Medical Publishers (P) Ltd, New Delhi, India, for accepting my thoughts for printing in a presentable form.

I am thankful to Dr HS Bhargava of M/s Scientific Literature Co., Indore, Madhya Pradesh, India, for his support and expert suggestions in the marketing of this book right from the beginning.

Last but not the least, I thank all the students of my college for their enthusiasm and positive response toward the subject of "communication skills", which has encouraged me to do more work in this field.

DISCLAIMERS

- India is a country with unity in diversity which embraces a variety of cultures, traditions, customs, and languages. Communication with any person is greatly influenced by these factors. So practically, it would be difficult for any author to write a single book on communication skills which fits with cultures and traditions of every part of our country. To make this book more practical, few Hindi sentences are included at several places. All of them are written in English fonts and are supported by their English translations. Similarly, readers may find a glimpse of cultures and traditions of central India at several places. They are requested to accept and modify them according to the language, cultures, and traditions of their place.
- Every medical student will become a doctor in future and every doctor is a student who is constantly learning the art of history taking. A major part of this book has been focused to the needs of medical students. Still, it includes many suggestions which would be more useful for the student in his future life when he would interact with the patients as a practicing doctor. Students are requested to interpret such suggestions accordingly.
- All names and cases, which have been mentioned in various examples in this book, are fictitious. Any resemblance with any living or dead person is purely coincidental.

Contents

Section 1: Doctor–Patient Communication

Chapter 1: Doctor–Patient Relationship   3
- Real Meaning of Good Communication Skills   3
- Levels of Doctor–Patient Communication   4
- Importance of History Taking   7
- Hazards of Poor Communication Skills   7

Chapter 2: What Does it Mean to be a Patient?   8
- Physical Stress   8
- Mental Stress   9
- Financial Stress   12

Chapter 3: An Approach to the Diagnosis   14
- Symptoms, Signs, and Diagnosis   14
- Importance of History Taking   18
- Role of Communication Skills   18
- Role of Investigations   19

Section 2: Foundation of Communication

Chapter 4: Basic Principles of Communication   27
- Process of Communication   27
- Basic Elements of Communication   28
- Various Types of Classification of Communication   31
- Common Channels of Communication   33
- Barriers of Communication   35

Chapter 5: Elements of Communication   39
- Description of Various Elements of Nonverbal Communication   42

Section 3: Format of Medical History

Chapter 6: What, Why, and How to Ask?   59
- Format of Medical History   61

Chapter 7: Patient's Profile   63
- Name   63
- Age   63
- Sex   65
- Residence   65
- Religion   66

- Occupation *67*
- Socioeconomic Status *69*

Chapter 8: Presenting Complaints — 70
- The Meaning of Presenting Complaints *70*

Chapter 9: History of Presenting Complaints — 81
- Elicitation of History of Presenting Complaints *86*

Chapter 10: Past History — 95
- General Considerations *95*
- History of any Significant Disease *96*
- History of Hospitalization *100*
- History of any Surgery *101*
- History of any Other Significant Event *102*
- History of Similar Complaints in Past *103*

Chapter 11: Personal History — 105
- General Considerations *106*
- Sleep *106*
- Appetite *107*
- Diet *109*
- Weight Change *110*
- Addiction *112*
- Bladder and Bowel Habits *116*
- Marital Status and Children *118*

Chapter 12: Family History — 119
- History of Contact *121*

Chapter 13: Menstrual and Obstetric History — 122
- Menstrual History *122*
- Obstetric History *127*

Chapter 14: Drug History — 129
- Commonly Used Drugs *130*
- Drugs for the Same Disease *130*

Chapter 15: Allergy History — 133

Chapter 16: Case History of Pediatric Patients — 135
- Format for Pediatric History *135*

Section 4: Student–Patient Interaction

Chapter 17: How to Take and Present a Case History? — 151
- Sufferings of a Patient *153*
- History Taking *153*
- Presentation of Case History *164*

Chapter 18: An Illustrated Case History — 167
- Presentation of Case History *173*

Section 5: Six Skills of Communication with Patients

Chapter 19: Listening Skills — 177

Chapter 20: Questioning Skills — 183
- Importance of Questioning in Communication *183*
- Selection of Relevant Questions *184*
- An Ideal Question *185*
- Why are You Asking? *185*
- Internal Feelings of the Patient *186*
- Types of Questions *188*
- Single Versus Multiple Questions *190*
- Extent of Enquiry *191*
- How to Improve Your Questioning Skills? *192*

Chapter 21: Answering Skills — 195

Chapter 22: Explanation Skills — 201

Chapter 23: Persuasion Skills — 215
- Hazards of Poor Persuasion Skills *216*
- How to Improve the Persuasion Skills? *218*
- How to Convince to Avoid? *221*

Chapter 24: Examination Skills — 224
- Role of Chaperon *225*
- Avoid Checking Old Documents in Beginning *226*

Index — *227*

Section 1

Doctor–Patient Communication

Section Outline

- Doctor–Patient Relationship
- What Does it Mean to be a Patient?
- An Approach to the Diagnosis

CHAPTER 1

Doctor–Patient Relationship

We get out of life what we put into it.
The way we treat others is the way we ourselves get treated.
—**Ben Carson**

Proper communication is the key to success in many professions. Medical profession is probably the best example of it. A doctor with immense knowledge and skills of his subject may not get the desired success if he is not communicating properly with his patient. In contrast, someone with average medical knowledge may impress his patients only because of his communication skills.

REAL MEANING OF GOOD COMMUNICATION SKILLS

It is generally considered that for a doctor to have *good communication skills* means to be kind, gentle, sympathetic, and polite with his patients. No doubt that these qualities are essential in medical profession, but a doctor cannot become successful only by being gentle and polite with his patients. In other words, the spectrum of the word communication skills is wrongly considered by many people to be limited to sympathy and politeness only. It is true that every patient expects his treating doctor to have these qualities. But above all, he wants his doctor to have following two qualities during communication:

1. He should look *interested* in listening to his patient's complaints
2. He should look *confident* while taking any decision for his patient's treatment.

If these two qualities (interested and confident) are missing in the doctor, most of the patients will prefer to switch over to some other physician for their treatment, even if the doctor is very gentle and polite.

Section 1: Doctor–Patient Communication

The relationship of doctor and patient is quite different from many other professions. Every person will be extremely cautious while selecting a doctor for his treatment because he knows that any error may lead to some irreversible damage to his body or life. He may not be very cautious in selecting a mechanic for repairing his bike or a plumber for sanitary fitting in his home because he knows that even if they commit a major mistake or negligence, it will never endanger his life or body.

Some medical students and doctors ignore the importance of training of communication skills, as they consider that they do not need it at all, simply because they are quite gentle and polite with their patients. There are several aspects of doctor-patient communication. Even if you are good in communication with your patients, it is always better to improve your skills to a higher level.

In short, a doctor can be considered to be having good communication skills if he is having following qualities:
- Decent appearance
- Gentle and polite in behavior
- Interested in listening to his patient's problems
- Confident while explaining him about the disease and its management.

LEVELS OF DOCTOR–PATIENT COMMUNICATION

The role of doctor-patient communication should not be considered limited to taking history of any patient. There are multiple levels where doctor is expected to have proper communication with his patient and family members. Let us understand it by imagining the following example:

"A woman visited to a doctor with complaint of pain in abdomen. After her examination, doctor advised her some investigations which revealed a tumor in her abdomen. It was removed surgically and was found to be highly malignant. Patient received full course of chemotherapy after surgery".

This looks like a typical case of standard management of some disease. Now, let us find the different levels where that doctor had to show his communication skills, in some or the other way, to the patient.

Level 1: Doctor took a proper history of the patient. He asked her several questions and listened to her complaints carefully.

Level 2: He performed her general and systemic (abdominal) examination gently but methodically and confidently.

Level 3: He explained her about the provisional diagnosis of her disease.

Level 4: He advised her some investigations and explained about their need.

Level 5: After few days, when the patient came back with the investigation reports, he explained her about the reports of investigations.

Level 6: Since, she was having an operable tumor, doctor persuaded her for the surgery by explaining its need, the possible complications of not removing the tumor, any alternative management, etc.

Level 7: At every level, she asked various types of questions to the doctor, which were answered by him confidently.

Level 8: The biopsy of removed tumor revealed it to be highly malignant. So, the doctor broke this bad news properly and explained her about the need of chemotherapy for its further management.

So, right from the beginning of the relationship, a doctor has to communicate with his patients (and their family members) at multiple levels in different ways. In other words, he can acquire good communication skill only if he has got following skills during communication with his patients:

a. *Questioning skills*: He should be able to ask specific questions in a form and language which is easily understood by the patient.
b. *Listening skills*: He should listen to patient's complaints attentively.
c. *Explanation skills*: He should explain him about the disease, its management plan, prognosis, etc.
d. *Persuasion skills*: He should be able to persuade his patient for some major intervention, such as hospitalization, surgery, etc.
e. *Answering skills*: He should give precise and confident answers to various types of questions from his patients.

It is essential for the doctor to have all of these skills during communication with the patient. Patient may not like to continue his treatment with some doctor who does not listen to him properly or who does not explain him about the disease adequately. These skills have been further elaborated in subsequent chapters of this book.

How do we Learn Communication Skills?

The three principle domains of learning of Bloom's taxonomy are cognitive, psychomotor, and affective. These can be simply understood as three H—Head, Hand, and Heart, respectively.

In medical science, the cognitive domain (Head) deals with the knowledge of normal and abnormal body system and functions. Student learns about them through various subjects of his syllabus, such as anatomy, physiology, pathology, surgery, etc. The psychomotor domain (Hand) is all about the manual skills, such as method of examination, making incision, suturing, dressing, etc. This is again learnt by the doctor during his student life, mainly during internship and postgraduation.

The affective (Heart) domain is all about the feeling and emotions. It makes the doctor gentle, kind, polite, and sympathetic to his patients. This involves the learning of proper ways of communication with patients at various stages. Unfortunately, this domain was not systematically covered in our education system for so many years. The major focus of the system was on methodical training of the other two domains and there was no systematic training of how to develop proper attitude for the patients. It was silently learnt by the students, mainly by *observing* their teachers and senior colleagues, during clinical postings, ward rounds, etc. (**Fig. 1.1**). Since, there was no

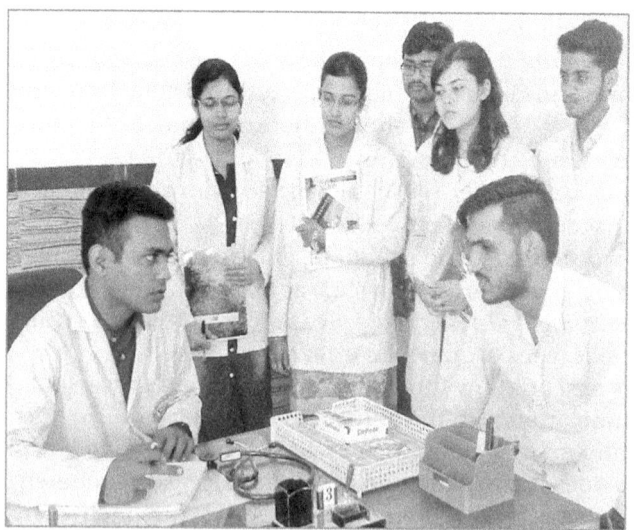

Fig. 1.1: Subconscious learning of communication.

formal training of communication skills, it was well said by someone that these skills were *caught and not taught*.

IMPORTANCE OF HISTORY TAKING

In almost all types of medical specialties, the communication of doctor and patient starts with a brief face-to-face conversation with each other. During this time, doctor first listens to his patient's problems, then asks him some questions, then examines him, and then explains him about his disease. The importance of this brief communication should not be underestimated by any doctor. Because during this period, doctor makes an assessment of his patient's disease and a patient does a simultaneous assessment of his doctor's communication skills. In fact, this short period of face-to-face conversation is a golden opportunity for the doctor to impress his patients by his good communication skills.

HAZARDS OF POOR COMMUNICATION SKILLS

Improper communication skills of the doctor will obviously lead to the dissatisfaction of the patient and his family members. The common reasons may be any one or more of the following:
- Doctor has probably not listened to my complaints properly
- He has not given me sufficient time and attention
- He has not examined me properly
- He has not explained me anything about my disease
- He was very casual while breaking this bad news to me
- He was not confident while telling me about this treatment.

An unsatisfied patient may be hazardous to the doctor in any of the following ways:
- He may visit some other doctor for a second opinion. This is probably the most common and unreported hazard of poor communication skills in medical profession. Many patients do not visit back to the doctor after their first consultation only because they are not satisfied with his communication skills.
- He may defame the doctor in his community and may not recommend him to any other patient.
- If the outcome of treatment is not favorable, an unsatisfied patient is more likely to take a legal action against his doctor.
- Unsatisfied patients and relatives are more likely to take some violent actions against the doctor and hospital.

CHAPTER 2

What Does it Mean to be a Patient?

Never forget that it is not pneumonia, but a pneumonic man who is your patient.
—**William Withy Gull**

At some or other time in our life, every one of us has undergone the bitter experience of being a patient. There is an endless list of diseases which effect one or more organ systems of human body. Some are acute, others are chronic. Some are mild, others are severe. But one fact is common that every disease brings some degree of turbulence in the routine life of every patient.

No one heartily wishes to visit to any hospital, neither as a patient nor as any relative of patient. There is only one time when people reach this place happily—the time of a new arrival in their family. Otherwise, there is always some major or minor problem, which has forcefully dragged them here.

It is essential for a doctor to deeply understand about the life and sufferings of any person, who has visited to him as his "patient". Different diseases affect different organs and present with different symptoms. But, all of them force the patient to go through a stressful period of his life. To understand deeply, this stress can be divided in following categories:

■ PHYSICAL STRESS

Human body is governed by a complex anatomy and physiology. Any kind of error in structure or functioning of any system will disturb its functioning to variable extent. Depending on the type and degree of this malfunctioning, patient will have different types of suffering, most of which are presented by him as chief complaints. For example, pain, weakness, fever, etc. None of them is pleasant or acceptable for him.

He only wants to get rid of them, as early as possible. This can be very well understood by imagining the life of some of the following patients:
- A man is having severe abdominal pain and vomiting because of acute pancreatitis.
- A man is unable to walk properly because of tuberculosis of hip joint.
- A woman with carcinoma esophagus is unable to swallow any solid food and is on liquid diet only.
- An old man is unable to see clearly because of cataract in his both eyes.

Unfortunately, most of the people judge the life of a patient mainly by his obvious complaints. To feel the real stress, one should try to look his life beyond the physical impact of his disease.

MENTAL STRESS

A disease effects not only the human body but the mind also. There are several factors related to the disease which bring a huge amount of mental stress to the patient and his family.

Why has it Happened to Me?

For many diseases, no obvious cause can be found. This leaves an unanswered question to the patient that why did it happen to him only. The cause is obvious when an alcoholic suffers from cirrhosis or pancreatitis, or a chronic smoker develops a lung cancer. But, the disease becomes even more painful when the patient is unable to find any obvious fault from his side. He can only blame it to his destiny. Following are some examples:
- A middle-aged man, who had always followed the principles of healthy lifestyle, developed a silent carcinoma of liver. By the time the first symptom arrived, it had already metastasized to his lungs.
- While playing in her school, a young girl suddenly felt acute pain in her abdomen, which was found to be because of acute appendicitis.
- A well-nourished and healthy child suddenly developed an inguinal hernia.
- A young man, who was driving his bike carefully, met with an accident, which broke several bones of his body.

This brings a special challenge to the doctor when any such patient asks him that why did it happen to him. No one is at fault here, neither the patient nor the doctor. It is his fate which has brought him in such position. Such questions should be handled carefully, with full sympathy toward the patient. He should be assured that he has not done anything wrong and everything is as per the wish of the God. He should be told about some other patients who had a worse destiny. For example, a surgeon explains the parents of a child with inguinal hernia as:

"Development of inguinal hernia is a natural phenomenon. There is no fault in your caring and no negligence on the part of his pediatrician. It is only because of his destiny, something which is beyond our control. In fact, I would say that he is lucky that you have quickly brought him here in this stage. Otherwise, some children come to us in a worse condition, with painful obstructed hernia."

You cannot change what has already happened to the patient. But, by pacifying him with such answers, you can at least make him think that he has got only some bad luck, and not the *worst*.

What Would be my Future?

As soon as the patient comes to know something abnormal with his body, a battery of questions starts hitting his mind. *What is it?... Will it get cured or not?... Will it need some surgery?... Is it something serious? ...Am I going to die?* And many more.

As the time passes, there occurs a continuous addition and deletion of questions in this questionnaire. He starts getting information about his problem from different sources, such as doctors, friends, relatives, internet, etc. Some information is good, others are bad. Some are authentic, others are fake.

> A 17-year-old girl incidentally noticed a small painless lump in her left breast. She got frightened, but was feeling hesitant in telling anyone in her family about it. She hoped that it may disappear in few days, but it did not. Round the clock, she started thinking about that lump only. After few days, with some hesitation, she decided to tell about it to a friend. Her friend told her about an old lady in her family who had recently died of breast cancer. This made the girl even more apprehensive. She searched about it on internet, but could not understand many words properly. Finally, she told about the lump to her mother. She took her to a surgeon. After examination, surgeon assured her and advised for FNAC of the lump. She could not sleep or eat properly, till the report had arrived. It was a benign fibroadenoma. Surgical excision was done after few days and everything went uneventful after that. But, the girl could never forget those days and nights of excessive apprehension and stress.

Different types of diseases bring mental stress of different degrees and varieties. Some diseases are obvious and clearly visible to the others (e.g., a lipoma on forehead region). Patient cannot ignore it mainly because of the cosmetic reasons and the constant comments from people around him (such as *what is it? how did it happen? why don't you show it to some doctor?,* etc.). Such comments obviously bring some amount of mental stress to him.

The Final Decision

Whenever you have to make some choice, it is bad when you have got too little options. But at the same time, it is worse to have too many options.

Soon after the detection of any problem, the major challenge for any patient is to make a firm choice from various options of its treatment. He starts searching for the best doctor, the best hospital, and the best possible treatment. Major problem arises when multiple options are available to him. He has to firmly select any one, which is not always an easy job. Sometimes, wanted or unwanted opinions from his friends and relatives may lead him to a state of confusion. If he decides to continue the treatment of one doctor, someone may ask him to consult some other doctor. Same problem occurs during the selection of hospital also. The good and bad experiences of various people with different hospitals confuse him badly.

> A 45-year-old man was diagnosed to be having a 15 mm stone in his right kidney. He consulted an urologist Dr A for it, who nicely explained him about the disease and its management plan. Patient readily agreed to get hospitalized for the endoscopic removal of stone after 2 days. Soon, his relatives came to know about his problem. His uncle called him and asked to take a second opinion from Dr B as Dr A had damaged one kidney of his friend. His son searched on internet and found that Dr C was the best urologist of the town. His friend advised him to not to go for surgery so early and to try some Ayurvedic treatment as his wife was totally cured by it. His neighbor warned him about the high charges and poor services of the hospital where he was planning to get himself operated. The poor man found himself in a state of big confusion, with multiple treatment options in front of him.

Another type of stress occurs when patient comes to know about the treatment plan of his disease, especially if it needs some major surgical procedure. Every patient wants to get rid of his suffering, as easily, as early, and as cheaply as possible. It is a natural instinct of any person to avoid any major inconvenience to his body or routine life. That is why many patients prefer to go for a second opinion, even if they are convinced with advice of their first doctor. Most of them silently hope for a miracle and expect some easier line of management from their second doctor.

Management of some diseases is universal and straightforward, every doctor in the world will follow the same line. For example, everyone will suture a fresh and deep wound; no one will try to heel it with some medicines. Similarly, if patient has got pedal edema due to renal failure, everyone will try to treat it conservatively; no one will aspirate or incise the patient's leg. But, in many other cases, there may be a difference of opinion of two doctors, and both of them may be correct. For example, a patient of intestinal obstruction was advised for immediate surgery by one surgeon, but the other surgeon preferred to keep him on conservative line for at least 24-48 hours. Here, both of them are having their own logics, and no one can confidently say that who is right and who is wrong. The first surgeon is afraid of complications of delay in surgery, while the second one is trying to save the patient from the complications of surgical exploration. There is a situation of dilemma and it is difficult for any doctor to take the decision with full confidence. *Does it need surgery? If yes, then should I do it now? Or, tomorrow?* This dilemma and difference of opinions further worsen the stress of the patient, whenever he tries to seek a second opinion for his problem.

FINANCIAL STRESS

More or less, every patient suffers from some degree of finacial loss because of his illness. The extent and impact of this loss varies from patient to patient. Broadly, this occurs in form of any one or both of the following reasons:
- Expenditures for investigations, medicines, hospitalization, doctor's charges, etc.
- Cessation of regular earnings from the occupation.

Whenever, it is about the expenditures on health and illness, many people of our country have to spend from their own pocket. Everyone is not covered under some insurance scheme. The amount to be spent can range from small to huge. Many a times, it is difficult for the doctor to predict the duration and expenditure of the treatment accurately. No doubt that the impact of this stress depends upon the financial status and reserves of the patient. Anticipating this problem, many people opt for the mediclaim policy. But sometimes, they get surprised to find that their disease is beyond the coverage of their mediclaim policy.

The second reason of financial loss is equally disturbing to the patient. As long as the patient is unable to perform his regular job, the income comes to a halt. People in service may get sick leave for few days, but not for a long period. The worst impact of this limitation occurs on the people who work on daily wages. They do not have a large financial reserve, and so, cannot afford to stay away from their work for more than few days.

What does a patient expect from his doctor?
Whenever a patient visits a doctor, he expects him to have some basic qualities. The outcome of any doctor-patient relationship largely depends upon the fulfillment of the expectations of patient. If he finds that his doctor is having most of the essential qualities, he continues his relationship with the doctor (such as by following his advices, visiting for follow-up, recommending other patients to him, etc.). In contrast, whenever he feels that the doctor is lacking some major qualities, he prefers to switch over to some other available doctor. Following are some of the basic expectations which are made by almost every patient during consultation with any doctor:

- He should be gentle and polite.
- He should listen to him attentively.
- He should examine him properly.
- He should explain him about the disease and plan of its management.
- He should speak in a language which is easily understood by the patient.
- He should look confident while speaking.
- He should not prescribe him unnecessary investigations or medicines.
- He should provide him an early and easy cure from his sufferings.
- He should be economic.
- He should be updated with the advanced knowledge of medical science.
- He should keep his information confidential.
- He should be easily approachable, especially during emergency conditions.
- He should refer him to the proper specialist, whenever required.

CHAPTER 3

An Approach to the Diagnosis

Symptoms are body's mother tongue. Signs are in foreign language.
—*John Brown*

Medical history of a patient is "the information obtained by asking specific questions to the patient, which help the physician in formulating a diagnosis and management plan for his disease".

It is also known as *anamnesis*, if the information is provided by patient himself. But if some other person informs about the disease of the patient (e.g., unconscious or uncooperative patient), it is called as *heteroanamnesis*.

Medical history of a patient can be obtained in following two forms:
1. *Comprehensive history taking*: A fixed and extensive set of questions is asked to every patient. This method is commonly used by the medical students.
2. *Iterative hypothesis testing*: Only limited and specific questions are asked to the patient, depending upon his/her disease. This method is commonly practiced by the consultants and practicing physicians.

SYMPTOMS, SIGNS, AND DIAGNOSIS

The term patient is derived from the Latin word *patiens* which means sufferance. So, the literal meaning of patient is "the one who suffers". To get remedy from his suffering, he visits a physician. The first target of the physician is to establish a *diagnosis* from the symptoms and the signs of his patient.

A symptom can be defined as—"an abnormal feature of a patient which is *complained* by the patient himself or by his relatives". For example, pain, vomiting, diarrhea, constipation, etc.

A sign can be defined as—"an abnormal feature of the patient which is noticed by the physician during his *examination*". For example, tenderness, fluctuation, crepitation, etc.

Symptoms are what the patient says while signs are what the physician sees (observes).

Some features may be a sign or a symptom depending on that *who has observed it first*. For example, a skin rash may be first noticed either by the physician (sign) or by the patient (symptom). In contrast, few features can exclusively be the symptoms as only the patient can experience them (e.g., pain, nausea, giddiness, etc.) while some others are exclusively signs as they can be detected only by the physician and not by the patient (e.g., fluid thrill, fluctuation, elevated blood pressure, etc.).

Whatever is complained by the patient to the physician cannot always be considered as a symptom. Only logical complaints should be recorded and presented as the symptoms. For example, if a patient says that *he is suffering from hernia*, it should not be considered as a symptom, as hernia is a diagnosis. Similarly, it is not uncommon to find the patients with palpitation and restlessness complaining the physician that their *blood pressure is raised*. Here, raised BP cannot be considered as a symptom, as it is a sign which can be detected only by the physician. Some of such unusual presentations of the complaints have been described in Chapter 8.

A physician seeks the diagnosis of disease on the basis of findings of case history and clinical examination of the patient. The first part (history taking) collects the "symptoms" of the patient while the second one (clinical examination) is all about the "signs".

Some symptoms indicate toward abnormalities of a particular system (e.g., hematuria indicates toward diseases of kidney, bladder, or urethra). In contrast, some other symptoms (such as abdominal pain, fever, etc.) are quite nonspecific and can be the presenting features of a large number of diseases from different systems of the body.

A disease can present with single or multiple symptoms (e.g., abdominal pain, vomiting, and fever occur in acute appendicitis). At the same time, a single symptom can be the presenting feature of multiple diseases (e.g., fever can be a presenting symptom of many diseases, such as malaria, typhoid, dengue, tuberculosis, etc.).

A list of diseases which present with similar symptoms is called as the *differential diagnosis* of that particular symptom. For example, "differential diagnosis of right iliac fossa pain" includes multiple diseases, such as acute appendicitis, right ureteric colic, acute mesenteric lymphadenitis, Meckel's diverticulitis, and many more. Differential diagnosis is commonly mentioned in reference to a symptom or to a diagnosis. For example, the above-mentioned list of diseases can also be called as the "differential diagnosis of acute appendicitis".

As soon as a patient complains of the first symptom to the physician, a list of probable differential diagnoses clicks in his mind. While asking various questions of the case history, a process of assessment runs in his brain simultaneously. It helps him in supporting any one and rejecting the others from the list. As the conversation proceeds, the list of differential diagnoses narrows down. For example, both Buerger's diseases and varicose veins can present with the complaint of chronic pain in lower limbs. Now, while interacting with any such patient, the physician keeps the possibility of both in his mind and seeks more information about his disease and lifestyle. These help him in selecting any one of them as the most probable diagnosis as:

- If the patient says that he is chronic smoker, his pain starts on walking for some distance and gets relieved by taking rest: these information go in favor of arterial insufficiency (Buerger's disease).
- But if he says that his occupation needs prolonged standing, his pain is maximum by the end of the day and he gets some relief on lying down and by elevating his limb: these information go in favor of venous incompetence (varicose veins).

So, even before examining his limb, the physician gets some idea of the probable diagnosis on the basis of information provided by the patient in his history (symptoms). Later on, he confirms it on the basis of findings of clinical examination (signs) and makes a clinical diagnosis of patient's disease.

It is the skill of a physician, which helps him to inquire about various symptoms by interrogating the patient and to detect various signs by conducting his proper clinical examination. By analyzing them together, he can identify what is troubling the patient. This diagnosis which is based only on the findings of medical history (symptoms) and clinical examination (signs) is known as "clinical diagnosis".

For example:

Symptoms: Abdominal pain, fever, and vomiting

Signs: Guarding and tenderness in right iliac fossa

Clinical diagnosis: Acute appendicitis

Chapter 3: An Approach to the Diagnosis

Once the clinical diagnosis is made, the physician sends the patient for suitable investigations, if required. The selection of investigations depends on the clinical diagnosis to a great extent. For example, two common acute abdominal conditions, *perforation peritonitis* and *acute appendicitis*, present with almost similar symptoms (such as abdominal pain, vomiting, fever, etc.), but the best diagnostic investigation for a case of perforation peritonitis is plain X-ray chest or abdomen (which shows free gas under diaphragm) while for acute appendicitis, it is abdominal ultrasound (which shows inflamed and distended appendix). This selection of appropriate investigation can be made only if the physician has made a correct clinical diagnosis by taking proper case history and by performing appropriate clinical examination of the patient. Otherwise, the patient will be unnecessarily subjected to useless investigations which will increase his financial expenditure.

Many a times, the clinical diagnosis made by a physician may get changed after subjecting the patient to appropriate investigations. Since, it is based only on symptoms and signs and is likely to be changed in future, it is also known as "provisional diagnosis" of the disease (dictionary meaning of *provisional*: arranged or existing for the present, likely to be changed later).

The diagnosis which is made on the basis of various investigation reports and after giving appropriate treatment to the patient is known as "final diagnosis" or "definitive diagnosis". For example, in the above-mentioned case of abdominal pain and tenderness in right iliac fossa:

Total leukocyte count: 16,000 cells/mm^3

USG of abdomen: Aperistaltic, noncompressible, and dilated blind tubular structure in right iliac fossa

Operative finding: Inflamed and enlarged appendix

Biopsy report: Ulcerated mucosal lining with heavy infiltration of polymorphonuclear cells in wall of appendix up to muscularis layer.

Final diagnosis: Acute appendicitis

The major task of a *medical student* is to make a clinical diagnosis on the basis of signs and symptoms. Beyond this, he can neither advise any investigation nor prescribe any treatment to the patient. However, he should have a proper theoretical knowledge of the investigations and treatment part of the disease. So, during his clinical training period, a student should mainly focus on developing skills of interrogating (for symptoms) and examining (for signs) the patients with different diseases.

IMPORTANCE OF HISTORY TAKING

History taking is an art and every doctor learns it throughout his life. First, he learns it from his teachers and then from his experiences.

It has been estimated that more than 80% of diagnoses in medical clinics can be made on the basis of history alone. While an appropriate history will guide the patient's management in proper direction, an incomplete or improper history may lead to unnecessary investigations and wrong treatment. Thus, a proper knowledge of the art of history taking is the key to success in medical practice.

Examination of a patient can only show the abnormalities present at the time of examination. On the other hand, his case history can also reveal multiple other aspects which are related to the development of his disease. For example, a gynecologist could not find anything abnormal in general, systemic, and gynecological examination of a female presenting with infertility. But when patient revealed a history of tuberculosis in her past, doctor started suspecting a diagnosis of tuberculous salpingitis, which is a common cause of female infertility in our country.

In short, the act of *history taking* is helpful to a physician in following ways:

- Symptoms help the physician in setting priorities of subsequent clinical examination of the patient. For example, if the patient is complaining of cough and breathlessness, his physician will pay more attention toward examination of his respiratory and cardiovascular systems, but the same physician will pay more attention on neurological examination of the patient presenting with ataxia and tremors.
- Symptoms and signs guide the physician in making a clinical diagnosis of patient's disease. This will help him in selecting the appropriate investigations for confirmation of the disease, if required.
- He can also assess the impact of disease on lifestyle of the patient.
- This short conversation helps him in judging the personality and intellectual level of his patient.
- Most importantly, this brief session of communication brings him an opportunity to gain the faith and confidence of his patient.

ROLE OF COMMUNICATION SKILLS

The role of history taking is much more than obtaining the information about the disease of the patient. This brief session of communication also brings an opportunity for the physician and the patient to make an assessment of each other's personality. During this conversation, a physician can make an evaluation of disease and the character of his patient (such as his behavior, intellectual level, etc.). At the same time, the patient makes an assessment of attitude of the physician toward him. By showing a gentle and confident attitude during communication, a doctor can very well gain faith and confidence of his patient.

A patient is always serious while selecting the suitable doctor for his disease as he knows that his wellness and life will be in his hands. In present era, due to the advancement of medical science, every city of our country has a large number of doctors of different specialities. This pool will keep on expanding in the future also. Nowadays, patients have got multiple options for treatment of any disease, ranging from economic to expensive and from experienced to young doctors. Along with so many other criteria, the *behavior* of the doctor also plays a major role in this selection. A doctor who is *gentle* and *confident* in his communication will certainly gain the faith of the patient and fame in his practicing area. One the other hand, a doctor with perfect knowledge and skill of his specialty may fail to succeed in his practice if he is not looking confident during communication with his patients. In such a case, the patient will never hesitate in switching over to some other doctor for treatment of his disease.

Theoretical knowledge and clinical skills of any doctor can be compared to some *cereals* (such as rice or wheat flour). By virtue of his knowledge alone, he can prepare some nutritious dish but that will not be palatable. Hence, he needs the *spices* of communication skills also. Only a proper combination of knowledge (cereals) and communication skills (spices) will lead to a nutritious and palatable recipe.

ROLE OF INVESTIGATIONS

Investigations are only supplementary to a proper clinical diagnosis.

The provisional diagnosis which is made on the basis of signs and symptoms is very much dependent upon the theoretical knowledge and examination skills of the doctor. Sometimes, it gets changed after subjecting the patient to various investigations and so, it is correctly called as a provisional diagnosis. The literal meaning of word "provisional" is something which is *serving only for the time being and which can be changed later*. For example:

> A 25-year-old male presented to a surgeon with complaints of severe pain in right iliac fossa region of abdomen, along with nonbilious vomiting. After his examination, the surgeon made a provisional diagnosis of *acute appendicitis* and sent him for basic investigations. His complete blood count was found to be in normal limits and urine examination showed microscopic hematuria. Ultrasonography of abdomen revealed normal appendix and a small stone in his right ureter. On this basis, his diagnosis was changed to *ureteric calculus* and the surgeon started his management accordingly.

> A 6-year-old child was brought to a pediatrician with complaint of severe pain in his right testicle since few hours. He initially suspected it to be case of *acute epididymo-orchitis*. But the Doppler ultrasonography revealed diminished blood flow in right testis, which shifted the diagnosis in favor of *testicular torsion*.

Many diseases present with almost similar signs and symptoms. So, this shift in diagnosis is a common phenomenon in routine clinical practice and even expert doctors are not always successful in making an accurate clinical diagnosis. Hence, before planning patient's definitive treatment, it is always better to get the relevant investigations done, if required. For example, in the above-mentioned case, though both appendicitis and ureteric stone can present with similar signs and symptoms, their management is completely different from each other. Appendicitis needs an urgent surgical intervention (open or laparoscopic) while ureteric stones are mainly managed either by conservative treatment or by endoscopic procedure. If the surgeon has made a wrong clinical diagnosis and has not confirmed it with appropriate investigations, further treatment will lead in a wrong direction and can be hazardous for the patient.

So, it is needless to say that investigations play an important part in the management of any disease. But at the same time, one should not forget that *the investigations are only supplementary to a proper clinical diagnosis*. Selection of appropriate investigation largely depends on the provisional diagnosis of the disease as described earlier in this chapter. A patient should be referred for the investigations only after taking a proper history and clinical examination. It would be a wrong method to send the patient for investigation directly without seeking the signs and symptoms of his disease.

Chapter 3: An Approach to the Diagnosis

A good physician always makes some provisional diagnosis before sending the patient to relevant investigations, but some others avoid it and directly send the patient for the series of investigations. For example, a patient with abdominal pain was advised for ultrasonography by the surgeon without doing a proper abdominal examination. Similarly, a patient with cough and breathlessness was straightway sent by the physician for an X-ray chest without performing a proper clinical examination of respiratory system. Once the patient comes back with the investigation reports, it becomes easier for them to make a diagnosis retrospectively. There can be several reasons behind this approach. Some may be afraid of making and writing a *wrong* provisional diagnosis on patient's case sheet. This fear is usually seen in postgraduation students in outpatient department (OPD) and clinical practitioners in early stages. Excessive bulk of the patients may be another reason which may prevent some doctors from performing proper interrogation and examination of the patient. No doubt that it looks like an easy and accurate method of diagnosing various diseases, but, in a long run, this habit may deteriorate the communication and examination skills of physician for various types of patients.

There is no substitute of proper history taking and clinical examination of the patient before sending him for investigations. Excessive dependency on investigations can be hazardous in the following ways:

- The interpretation of various common investigations largely depends on the expertise of the person performing them (e.g., pathologist, radiologist, etc.) and also on the quality of machines used. Occasionally, there can be some error in the reports even from the most experienced persons. If a doctor totally relies on them and fails to perform interrogation and examination of the patient before or after receiving the reports, a wrong interpretation would definitely lead the treatment in a wrong direction. For example:

> A 45-year-old patient presented to a surgeon with complaints of abdominal pain and vomiting. Without eliciting detailed history and performing proper examination, he advised him for X-ray and ultrasonography of abdomen. Both the investigations could not find anything abnormal and so, he sent him home after prescribing some antibiotics and analgesics. After 2 days, patient reported back in emergency with features of perforation peritonitis, which was secondary to the rupture of inflamed appendix.

This error happened here because the radiologist was not able to find the features of inflamed appendix in ultrasonography. This problem is more common in cases of ultrasonography as compared to X-rays, CT scans, magnetic resonance imaging (MRI), etc., as in other cases, proper *film* is available (along with the report) to the doctor to suspect some abnormality.

The knowledge and skill of making appropriate clinical diagnosis also helps the physician in challenging the investigation report (both false positive and false negative) in some cases. For example:

> An 11-year-old child presented to a surgeon with a palpable lump in his abdomen since few days. He was also having the report of his abdominal sonography, which had reported his lump as some tumor arising from his retroperitoneum. The lump was hard, nontender, and freely mobile. Child was also having a complaint of chronic constipation. Surgeon's mind was not going in favor of the sonological diagnosis. Instead of proceeding ahead with the same, he preferred to repeat the investigation. The lump was found to be a fecaloma (impacted hard mass of feces) in his sigmoid colon.

- As mentioned earlier, clinical diagnosis helps the doctor in selecting the most appropriate investigation for a particular patient. Otherwise, the patient will be subjected to a large number of unnecessary investigations. This will not only increase the *financial burden* on him, but may also expose him to the risks of *investigation hazards* [e.g., radiation exposure in X-ray and CT-scan, allergy to contrast agent in intravenous pyelogram (IVP), etc.]. Besides, in case of an acute and emergency problem, these useless investigations will waste the precious *time* and will unnecessarily delay the commencement of proper management of the patient. For example:

> Two poor patients presented to a surgeon with similar complaints of abdominal pain and vomiting. After taking proper history and performing methodical examination, he was able to make a provisional diagnosis of acute appendicitis for case 1 and intestinal obstruction for case 2. So, he advised abdominal ultrasonography for first patient and X-ray abdomen for the second one. This saved their precious time as well as the financial expenditure.

Chapter 3: An Approach to the Diagnosis

- Sometimes, investigations may detect some different problem which may divert the management to a totally different direction. For example:

> A 50-year-old chronic smoker presented with complaints of abdominal pain and occasional vomiting. Ultrasonography of abdomen revealed some stones in his gallbladder. The surgeon failed to take proper history and examination both before and after getting the investigation reports. All symptoms were attributed to gallstones and so, his cholecystectomy was performed, but the patient continued to suffer from same complaints even after removal of his gallbladder. Further examination and investigations revealed that he was suffering from peptic ulcer disease. Gallstones were asymptomatic and incidentally detected in ultrasonography.

- Advising an unnecessary investigation without proper indication can be hazardous to the reputation of the doctor also. Patients always prefer a physician who makes an accurate diagnosis on basis of minimum possible number of investigations. In a long run, a tendency of prescribing too many investigations may defame a physician in his practicing area.

Occasionally, some patients come with half knowledge of their disease, which is mostly obtained either from internet surfing or by discussing with some other patient. So, they may insist the doctor to advise them some specific investigation. Instead of accepting their choice, doctor should rather try to convince them about the necessity, advantages, and hazards of various investigations. For example:

> A rich patient was too much worried for his health. Once, he visited to a young physician with complaint of weakness and loss of appetite. He insisted the doctor to advise him all available investigations, without thinking about the expenditure. Since, symptoms were vague and nonspecific, the young inexperienced doctor prescribed him a large number of investigations. As expected, almost all of the reports were absolutely normal. Later on, patient visited several other doctors for his problem. Everyone was amazed to find the bulk of reports of useless and nonindicated investigations.

Investigation of choice should be the investigation of physician's choice and not of patient's choice.

- Excessive dependency on investigations may also affect the communication and examination skills of the doctor. In a long run, he may find difficulty in making a clinical diagnosis of even common diseases, if the desired investigations are not available. It has been estimated that more than 80% diagnoses in medical clinics can be made on the basis of history alone. It should be always remembered that there is no substitute of proper history taking and good clinical examination. Investigations are only supplementary to a proper clinical diagnosis. They should be advised judiciously only after taking the best possible efforts to make some clinical diagnosis of the disease.

Section 2

Foundation of Communication

Section Outline

- ❖ Basic Principles of Communication
- ❖ Elements of Communication

CHAPTER 4

Basic Principles of Communication

If you listen carefully to the patients, they will tell you the diagnosis.
—*Sir William Osler*

Proper communication is the key to success in many professions. Medical profession is probably the best example of it. Hence, it is essential for every medical student and doctor to know about the minute details of the process and elements of communication. No doubt that proper knowledge of the subject is quite important in any profession. But, even the best knowledge of a doctor may fail to impress and satisfy his patients, if he is not aware of the appropriate skills of communication.

PROCESS OF COMMUNICATION

The simplest definition of communication is *an exchange of any message between two or more people.* This message can be in form of spoken or written words, or as some expression or gesture.

The process of communication can be easily understood by imagining following example **(Fig. 4.1)**.

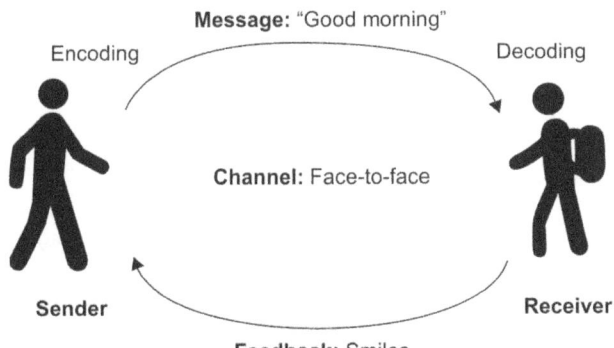

Fig. 4.1: Process of communication.

On his morning walk, Mr S sees Mr R on the other side of the road. He smiles and says politely "Good morning" to Mr R. In its response, Mr R smiles and waves his hand toward Mr S.

Now, this communication process requires following elements and actions:

- *Sender:* He is the person who has got some message for transmission in his mind. Also known as Encoder or Transmitter (Mr S).
- *Receiver:* He is the person who receives the message from the sender. Also known as Decoder (Mr R).
- *Message:* It is the major message which is to be transmitted by sender to the receiver. This can be in verbal or nonverbal form (In this example: Good morning).
- *Encoding:* This is the process of framing the message in the language and form which are easily understood by the receiver (In this example, Mr S framed his message in English language and spoke it in a polite tone with a smile on his face).
- *Channel:* This is the medium through which message is transmitted from the sender to the receiver. Some common channels of communication are face-to-face conversation, telephonic conversations, written texts, etc. (In this example, Face-to-face conversation).
- *Decoding:* This is the process of understanding verbal and nonverbal elements of the message by the receiver. Spoken messages are decoded by the act of hearing, while written messages are decoded by reading (In this example, Mr R *heard* the words "Good morning" and polite tone from Mr S and also, *saw* the smile on his face.).
- *Feedback:* This is the response given by the receiver to the sender, immediately after receiving the message. Like the original message, the feedback can be in both verbal and nonverbal forms (In this example, Mr R did not speak any word, but he smiled and waved his hand toward Mr S).

BASIC ELEMENTS OF COMMUNICATION

The message, which is transmitted from sender to receiver, can be divided in following three components:
1. *Verbal:* This includes the "words" of message, which are transmitted in spoken or written form.
2. *Paraverbal:* This includes various elements of paralanguage, such as speed, pitch, tone, volume, use of pause, stress, etc.

3. *Nonverbal:* This includes some important elements, such as gestures, facial expressions, eye contact, etc.

These three elements are also called as three "V"s of communication: Verbal, Vocal (Paraverbal), and Visual (Nonverbal).

During *face-to-face conversation*, all three components are transmitted from sender to receiver. Because, both sender and receiver can listen as well as see each other. In contrast, during *telephonic conversation*, verbal and paraverbal elements become more important as there is no nonverbal communication between sender and receiver, as they cannot see each other. Similarly, *written texts* (letters, e-mails, messages, etc.) carry only verbal elements (words), provided that no special feature, such as bold fonts, emoticons, etc., are used.

The impact of these three elements during communication can be easily understood by doing a simple experiment. When you watch some movie on television, you receive and successfully decode all three elements from various characters, i.e., words (verbal), tone (paraverbal), and body language (nonverbal). Now, switch over to some movie which is in a language which is not understood by you. Now you will be able to decode only tone and body language of its characters, as the spoken words will not be understood by you. In next step, turn off the volume of your television set. At this stage, you will try to interpret the activities only on the basis of body language of different characters of that movie, as you cannot hear their words and tone.

A blind person interprets the conveyed message only on the basis of verbal and paraverbal elements, as he cannot see the nonverbal activities of the sender. In contrast, a deaf person tries to interpret the conveyed message only on the basis of body language, as he cannot hear the spoken words and voice tone.

It has always been a matter of great curiosity to know that how much contribution is made individually by these three elements in transmitting any message during face-to-face conversation. The famous anthropologist Ray Birdwhistell believed that only one third of any message is conveyed through the spoken words. Albert Mehrabian, a clinical psychologist, stated that during face-to-face conversation, whenever there is any exchange of emotions and feelings, only 7% of message is transmitted by spoken words. The remaining 93% transmission is through paraverbal (38%) and nonverbal (55%) elements. This is known as 7-38-55 rule, which clearly indicates that verbal element gives the least contribution during face-to-face communication. In other words, how you say something is more important than what you say.

Systematic research on the role of nonverbal communication and behavior was started by Charles Darwin through his book *"The

Expression of Emotions in Man and Animals" (1872). He believed that this type of communication has been acquired by the human through the process of evolution, as it is the only way of communication amongst animals. For example, some animals make a peculiar expression to threaten their enemy by exposing their canines.

Verbal communication is largely conscious, while nonverbal communication is largely subconscious. Both paraverbal and nonverbal elements are encoded (by sender) and decoded (by receiver) subconsciously.

Sometimes, we perform nonverbal communication deliberately, either to reinforce or substitute the verbal message. For example, if you are wishing 'All the best' to your friend before his exam, you will look more concerned if you also raise your thumb simultaneously. Here, the nonverbal act of raising the thumb is augmenting the verbal element of spoken words. Similarly, in some cases, when it is not possible to communicate verbally, nonverbal messages are used to replace the words completely, e.g., raising your thumb to wish your friend on stage, or waving your hand to call the waiter in a crowded noisy restaurant, etc.

Whenever, there is a mismatching between the verbal and nonverbal elements of any message, our brain predominantly decodes the nonverbal elements. In other words, the impact of paraverbal and nonverbal elements is much more than the literal meaning of spoken words. This can be understood by imagining that in the above example, Mr S says "Good morning" to Mr R in a harsh tone and with angry looks on his face. Here, the spoken words are same (Good morning), but now Mr R will decode and interpret the message in a different way and will give a totally different type of feedback (e.g., amazed or angry, etc.) to Mr S. Such messages, in which verbal and nonverbal elements contradict each other, are also known as mixed messages.

Now, let us consider these rules in relation to the medical profession with the help of following examples:

> A female patient was explaining about her disease to the doctor. While listening to her problems, doctor was not maintaining proper eye contact with her. For majority of time, he was looking at some object on his table. He was leaned backward on his chair with blank expressions on his face. Also, he never nodded his head while listening, nor did he produce some vocal cue or any comment in response to her speech. Though he was attentively listening to all of her problems, still she felt that the doctor was not interested in knowing more about her disease. So, she switched over to some other doctor for her treatment.

Chapter 4: Basic Principles of Communication

> A middle-aged patient was having complaints of abdominal pain and vomiting. His ultrasonography revealed multiple stones in his gallbladder. He visited to a young surgeon, who told him that his disease will require surgical removal of gallbladder. But, while explaining him about his disease, surgeon was speaking in a very low voice. He had kept his both hands in his pockets and was not maintaining proper eye contact with the patient. This raised some doubt in the mind of the patient about the confidence and capability of surgeon, and so, he immediately visited a senior surgeon to take a second opinion.

It is interesting to notice that during face-to-face conversation, a person can receive a message from the other person through any one or more of his four senses:
1. *Auditory:* By listening the spoken words (verbal) and various paraverbal elements associated with them (such as tone, volume, etc.)
2. *Visual:* By observing various elements of body language, such as posture, gesture, facial expressions, etc.
3. *Olfactory:* The smell of various elements, such as perfume, deodorant, after shave, etc., also gives some pleasant or unpleasant sensation to the receiver.
4. *Tactile:* During communication, the simple act of touching by a person to the other person also conveys some kind of positive or negative message.

VARIOUS TYPES OF CLASSIFICATION OF COMMUNICATION

In our routine life, communication is an essential process which occurs contineously in various forms. There are several ways in which this process can be classified and understood:
1. *Models of communication* **(Fig. 4.2):**
    a. Transmission model: This can be simply called as a one way communication. There is no interchange of position between sender and receiver, i.e., sender is always a sender and receiver is always a receiver. Also, there is no instant feedback from receiver to sender. Common examples are messaging through television, radio, newspaper, etc.
    b. Transactional model: In this model, although only one person plays the role of sender, but along with sending the message, he

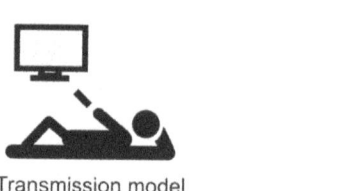

Fig. 4.2: Models of communication.

simultaneously receives an instant feedback from the receiver. This type of communication occurs during lectures, public speaking, etc. One person continuously sends message to the audience. But at the same time, he continuously receives their feedback through their nonverbal communication, such as facial expressions, gestures, etc.
  c. Interaction model: This is a model of two-way communication. There is continuous interchanging of position between sender and receiver. For some time, one person speaks and the other one listens. After that, speaker becomes the listener and listener becomes the speaker, and the process goes on. Majority of communication between a doctor and the patient occurs through this model. A doctor has to play the role of a speaker as well as a listener, and so, he should have a good command on both the speaking and listening skills.
2. *Formal versus informal communication:*
  a. Formal communication: This type of communication occurs in a well set environment. Both sender and the receiver have to follow certain preset rules. For example, communication during office meetings, lectures, seminars, etc.
  b. Informal communication: There is only some casual talk amongst the people, without following any fix rules. For example, communication during social parties, friends' meetings, family get-together, etc.
3. *Depending on the number of individuals:*
  a. One-to-one communication: There is only one sender and one receiver. For example, communication between doctor and a patient.

b. Small group communication: One person has to communicate with multiple receivers, e.g., communication between family members, friends, etc.
c. Public communication: One person addresses to a large number of persons, e.g., during public speech. This type of communication follows the transaction model of communication.
d. Mass communication: One way communication through media, such as television, radio, newspaper, website, etc. This follows the transmission model of communication.

In medical profession, majority of communication of the doctor occurs as a one-to-one (with patient) or small group (with patient and his family members) communication.

COMMON CHANNELS OF COMMUNICATION

In our routine life, the process of communication occurs though various types of channels. Following is the description of some of the common channels of communication (**Fig. 4.3**):

- *Face-to-face conversation:* This is the most common channel of communication in our routine life. It transmits all three elements of communication (verbal, paraverbal, and nonverbal) from sender to the receiver. In medical profession, almost all communication between a doctor and the patient occurs through this channel.
- *Telephonic conversation:* This mode of communication has become common since last few decades only. Only verbal and paraverbal elements are transmitted, as both sender and receiver cannot see each other on a voice call.
- *Written text:* This can be in form of the letters, e-mails, text messages, etc. Unless some special highlighting is used, this channel simply transmits only the verbal (as written words) component of message. Still, the sender can make some extra emphasis by highlighting some part of the text by special features, such as capital letters, underlining, bold fonts, etc.

All three channels have got different merits and demerits. For example, written texts do not transmit anything more than plane words. But at the same time, they can preserve the message for indefinite time. In contrast, unless there is any audio or video recording, the message of face-to-face and telephonic conversation cannot be preserved or repeated in future.

Section 2: Foundation of Communication

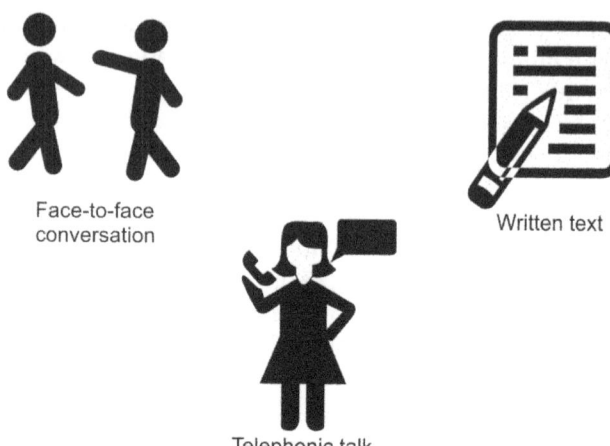

Fig. 4.3: Common channels of communication.

It is very important for the sender to select the most appropriate channel to convey the message. For example, it will be better if a teacher greets his student "good morning" by face-to-face conversation rather than by writing "good morning" on the board. Face-to-face communication is best for the messages where the emotions and feelings play an important role, e.g., explaining about the prognosis to the patient. In contrast, if the message is long and it is difficult for the receiver to remember it only through verbal instructions, it will be better to convey it through written texts, e.g., brochure explaining the exercises and dietary instruction.

Importance of Feedback

Feedback is the response given by the receiver to the message from the sender. Feedback is the mirror of communication. It is like an acknowledgment given by the receiver that he has received the message.

Like the message of the sender, the feedback of receiver can be of both verbal and nonverbal types. For example, during face-to-face communication, the receiver can give an instant feedback to the sender either by some words or by some gestures (head nodding), facial expressions (such as smile, surprised, confused, etc.) or as a combination of both.

Chapter 4: Basic Principles of Communication

Receiver can give his feedback either spontaneously (such as head nodding, vocal cues, facial expressions, etc.) or on being asked by the sender (such as *"Is it clear to you?", "Have you understood it properly?"*, etc.). It is always better to confirm the understanding of message by asking such questions, especially after some long or important message.

During communication in clinical practice, sender (doctor) should keenly notice the feedback of the receiver (patient). It will guide him to decide the adequacy and appropriateness of communication.

> A doctor was explaining his patient about his disease and its management (such as medicines, diet, precautions, etc.). While explaining, he noticed that the patient was nodding his head intermittently. But, while listening about the medicines, patient stopped nodding his head and gave some expression of confusion. This was noticed by the doctor. So, he asked the patient – *"Have you understood about the medicines properly?"* Patient accepted that he was unable to understand some instructions. Doctor explained him again in a slightly different way. Then he asked the patient to tell him back all the instructions. This time, patient had clearly understood everything, and so, he was able to reflect it back to the doctor properly.

BARRIERS OF COMMUNICATION

A barrier can be simply defined as anything which interferes in proper communication between two or more persons. Following are some of the common barriers during face-to-face communication, especially in context of doctor-patient communication.

- *Physical barrier:* This can be in form of noise, poor illumination, distance, etc.

  It is quite annoying to communicate with someone in a noisy surrounding. Noise interferes with the proper hearing of the spoken messages. During communication with patients, some common sources of noise can be the surrounding crowd, noisy fan, television in waiting room, etc. Moreover, presence of several unrelated persons in surrounding may sometimes make the patient hesitant in communicating with his doctor properly (e.g., in casualty, busy wards, etc.).

  Adequate illumination is essential for proper face-to-face communication. It helps both sender and receiver in watching each other's facial expressions. Moreover, sometimes it also helps the person in understanding the spoken words by watching the lip movements of the speaker, especially if he/she is speaking in a very low volume.

Similarly, if the surrounding atmosphere is uncomfortable for doctor or patient or both (such as hot, humid, suffocating, etc.), they may not be able to communicate with each other comfortably after some time.

- *Language barrier:* Language is the greatest power for communication amongst human beings. But, if not used properly, it can become the greatest barrier also.

  For success of any communication, it is obviously essential that the language used by the sender should be well understood by the receiver. Even a single word of some different language may make the whole message difficult for the receiver. Either he may not understand it, or may misinterpret it for some other word. This can happen if the doctor is casually using some difficult words (such as English words, medical terminologies, etc.) during communication with the patient. Similarly, sometimes patient may use some local terminology for any symptom or disease, which may be quite new and strange for the doctor.

  > An intern was taking history of a rural patient in medicine OPD. While asking about the bladder and bowel habits, he carelessly used the word *toilet*. Though the patient could not understand its meaning, still he also carelessly responded that he was not having any problem with his *toilet*. Also, he gave a past history of his surgery for some malignant abdominal tumor. The intern was surprised to know that the patient had applied *hot fomentation* over his abdomen after surgery. Actually, patient had told him that he had received *sikaai* after his abdominal surgery. This word literally means hot fomentation, but is popularly used for *radiotherapy* by many rural patients.

- *Cultural barrier:* Some elements of communication are greatly influenced by culture and are variable in different countries, such as eye contact, physical touch, interpersonal distance, etc. This barrier becomes significant when persons from two different culture or countries communicate with each other.

Chapter 4: Basic Principles of Communication

> During face-to-face communication, the interpersonal distance is much shorter in Italy than in Australia. Because of this reason, an Italian and an Australian person may feel uncomfortable during face-to-face communication with each other. Australian will not be comfortable when Italian will stand very close to him. At the same time, Italian may feel that Australian is not interested in communicating with him, only because of his distance from him. Here, both persons are following the practices of their own culture. But, the barrier is occurring merely because of the differences in cultures. Similar problem may also occur with some other elements, such as touching, eye contact, etc.

Practically, this barrier is rarely faced during the routine communications between doctor and patients, as both of them mostly belong to the same culture and country.

- *Mental barrier:* The internal thought process of the doctor imparts a significant effect on the quality of his communication with patients. A tired and exhausted doctor (e.g., at the end of a busy OPD, after some long surgery, etc.) may not be able to communicate with his patients properly. His physical or mental fatigue may act as a significant barrier for the proper communication.

Sometimes, a preoccupied thinking about the personality of some patient may create some degree of barrier in communication. By virtue of his experience, doctor may judge a patient too early. This phenomenon is known as stereotyping. For example, he may believe that the, *mothers are always over conscious about their child, females always exaggerate their complaints, old people talk mostly about irrelevant matters,* etc. Many a times, this judgment may be totally wrong.

Similarly, many a times doctors do not allow the patient to speak completely as *they already know that what he is going to say*. For example, during season of some viral infection, if a doctor gets a series of patients with similar complaints (such as fever, malaise, body ache, etc.), he may start examining the patient or prescribing the investigation or treatment even before patient finishes his complaints. Sometimes, this premature termination of communication may result in missing of some important information.

Another type of mental barrier occurs when the doctor *thinks of something else* while listening to the patient. This is known as internal distraction. Externally, he may look, such as listening to the patient. But, internally, he may be thinking about something else, such as thinking about the next question to be asked, about some other patient, about some other important works, etc. These thoughts may distract his mind from listening to the patient attentively.

- *Miscellaneous barriers:* Following are some more examples of uncommon but significant barriers for proper doctor-patient communication:
  - Selection of proper channel is quite important during communication. Face-to-face communication is best for conveying the messages with some feelings and emotions. But, this channel may not be appropriate for some complex and lengthy messages. For example, a patient may forget if his doctor gives him multiple dietary instructions verbally, such as *what-to-eat* and *what-not-to-eat*. It may be difficult for him to preserve and recall the same instructions later. So, it will be better for both doctor and the patient if such complex instructions are communicated in form of written texts (such as handwritten prescription, printed brochures, etc.). In contrast, it will be better if the doctor explains about the common complications of disease or treatment through direct face-to-face conversation with patient, rather than informing him about them through some printed brochure.
  - Illegible handwriting of doctor in his prescription may act as a barrier of proper text communication with his patients, pharmacists or the other doctors.

CHAPTER 5

Elements of Communication

> *The single biggest problem in communication is the illusion that it has taken place.*
> —George Bernard Shaw

The three basic elements of communication (verbal, paraverbal, and nonverbal) are often abbreviated as 3 Vs—Verbal, Vocal, and Visual, respectively. Following is the detailed description of the individual element:

Verbal

The verbal element forms the principle content of the message, which is transmitted through spoken or written form. During communication, it is very important for the sender to take care of the understanding of the receiver. He should avoid using the words which may not be understood (or may even be misunderstood) by the receiver.

To understand the importance of language, readers are requested to reply the following question instantly:

"Have you taken your frukost today?"

If you could not give an instant reply, let us give it another chance:

"Have you taken your breakfast today?"

Frukost is a Swedish word, which means breakfast in English.

In this example, a single word (breakfast) from a well-known language (English) was replaced to a translated word in an unknown language (Swedish). This small change had converted a very simple question to a very difficult one.

The same problem is faced by the receivers when the sender uses a language which is unknown for them. For example, if a doctor uses multiple English words or medical terminologies, all of his patients may not be able to understand his question or instructions.

Sender can easily perceive the intellectual level and understanding of the receiver during initial few moments of the communication. Then, he should choose his words accordingly.

It is interesting to know that during doctor–patient communication, there are several occasions when the use of some unconventional words makes the communication even better. Some diseases, procedures, or objects are popularly known by some specific names by the native people. These words are more commonly used by rural and low socioeconomic class people. The list of such words is vast and varies from place to place. For example, at some places, tubectomy, hysterectomy, and radiotherapy are known as *chhota operation* (English meaning: small operation), *bada operation* (English meaning: big operation), and *sikaai* (English meaning: hot fomentation), respectively. Now, instead of using the words of standard language (such as Hindi, English, etc.), it will be better if the doctor uses these well-known words for communication with the suitable patients.

In short, same language may not be appropriate for communication with all types of patients. A doctor must learn to modify his language according to the understanding of his patients.

The importance of language should not be ignored even during writing some instructions on patient's prescription. The important instructions about medicines, diet, precautions, etc., should be clearly written in the language which is easily understood by the patient.

Apart from the selection of words, brevity and clarity are two important components of verbal communication. Sender should be able to convey the important message in minimum possible words (brevity), as it may become very difficult for the receiver to understand and retain long messages. Similarly, the spoken words should be pronounced clearly (clarity), otherwise the receiver may not be able to understand some part or whole of the message.

Apart for communication with patients, it is also important to take care of selection of words while communicating with your colleagues in front of the patients, e.g., during bedside conversation. As far as possible, some words with dual meaning (such as sex, drugs, etc.) should be avoided. Similarly, sometimes, it is better to converse with your colleagues in a language which is not understood by the patient. The well-known words should be replaced by the medical terms, such as hypertension for high BP, malignancy for cancer, etc. Otherwise sometimes, patient and his relatives may misinterpret the conversation.

Chapter 5: Elements of Communication

During his routine round in the ward, a consultant started discussing about the disease of a patient near his bed. Patient was from low socioeconomic class and conversation was going on in English language. At the end of whole discussion, the consultant told his residents—"Luckily, he is not having any cancer, otherwise it would have been a highly serious condition". Patient was having some benign and curable tumor, but he and his wife became very anxious after this bedside conversation because they both could understand only two words from the whole discussion: *cancer* and *serious*.

Paraverbal

The paraverbal communication is made by the sender through various elements, such as speed, tone, volume, pitch, pause, stress, etc. These are also known as the elements of *paralanguage*, as they are spoken out, but still they are not the true words. A systematic study of the effect of these elements in communication is known as *vocalics*.

Some of these elements are described below, especially in context of communication with patients:

- *Speed* - A typical speaker speaks about 100–125 words in a minute. It should be remembered by the doctor that while he is speaking, the patient is trying to understand his spoken words. Hence, he may miss some important message if the speed is too fast. Speed should be moderate, neither too fast, nor too slow.
- *Volume* - Just like the speed, the volume should also be moderate, neither too low, nor too loud. Words spoken with very low volume may not be clearly heard by the patients. At the same time, no patient would like his doctor to converse with him in loud voice, as he may not like the others to hear about his problem. Doctor should speak to his patient in moderate volume, which should be further reduced while talking about some personal matters, such as sexual history, addiction, etc.
- *Tone* - During communication with patients, tone of the doctor should be gentle and soft. While explaining or instructing the patient, his tone should be of adult-to-adult sharing type and not of parent-to-child type.
- *Pause* - It is very impressive to use pauses of adequate length at several places of the speech, as used by politicians, motivational speakers, etc. Pause is usually taken after some important point, as it gives the listener some moments to think over it.
- *Stress* - Just like pause, some extra emphasis on any part of message can be given by speaking it with some stress. For example, following is a simple instruction given by a doctor to his patient:

"You will not be able to eat anything for 4 hours after your surgery".

The impact of this message can be increased by giving extra stress on some important words. It will be taken more seriously by the patient if the doctor puts some stress on words, such as *anything* and *4 hours*.

In short, a simple monotonous message can be made more meaningful and impactful by taking proper care of various paraverbal elements, such as tone, stress, pause, etc.

Nonverbal

As described earlier, this is the strongest and most impactful element during face-to-face conversation between two or more persons. This is popularly known as the "body language", but both of them are quite different. Body language is mainly manifested by movement of some part or whole of the body (e.g., by gait, gesture, etc.) while nonverbal communication includes body language plus other elements, such as appearance, possessions, etc.

■ DESCRIPTION OF VARIOUS ELEMENTS OF NONVERBAL COMMUNICATION

Unlike verbal element, nonverbal elements are mainly encoded and decoded subconciously. Following is the description of some of these elements, especially in context of doctor-patient communication :

Personal Appearance

Some researchers state that it takes only a fraction of a second for our mind to get an idea about the character and personality of a person by his appearance. This impression, which is popularly known as the first impression, becomes more firm in next 3 seconds.

The appearance of a person is determined not only by his facial appearance. It includes several other elements, such as clothing, possessions, etc. A systematic study of the impact of clothing and other objects on personality and nonverbal communication of a person is known as *artifactics* or *objectics*.

All over the world, medical profession is considered to be a noble profession and so, the appearance and first impression of any doctor will play a major impact on the overall outcome of the doctor–patient communication. In several studies, it was found that the majority of patients prefer to see their doctor (male or female) in formal attire, instead of the casual attire. Similarly, the impact of various possessions,

Chapter 5: Elements of Communication

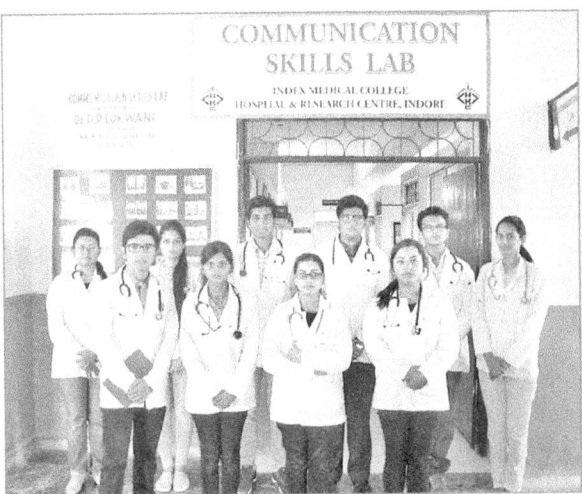

Fig. 5.1: Descent appearance suits medical profession.

such as shoes, belt, jewelry, pen, etc., should not be ignored. Just like the dressing, these items should be decent and should match with the dignity of our profession (**Fig. 5.1**).

> A child met an accidental head injury at his home. His parents took him urgently to a nearby hospital. A young doctor examined the child and advised for his hospitalization. Parents noticed that the doctor was wearing a faded and torn jeans, T-shirt, and sport shoes, with an apron on his shoulder. He was around 25-year-old, with a large tattoo on his right arm. Though he was quite competent and capable to manage such cases, still the parents preferred to take their child to some other hospital.

It is well said by someone that the first impression is the last impression. It provides a halo effect during further communication, i.e., a positive impression of someone gives you a positive feeling about his other characters also. In contrast, if the first impression is negative, it becomes very difficult to cover up this loss during subsequent communication.

Posture

It can be simply defined as the position in which the person keeps his body during sitting or standing. In our routine life, almost all of our communication occurs in any of these two positions. Following

are certain positive suggestions to improve your posture during communication:
- Keep your spine straight and chin slightly up. Avoid slouching, side tilting, or backward tilting (**Fig. 5.2**)
- While listening to someone in sitting position, bend slightly forward (Sprinter's position). This will give the person a feeling that you are interested in listening to him (**Fig. 5.3**).

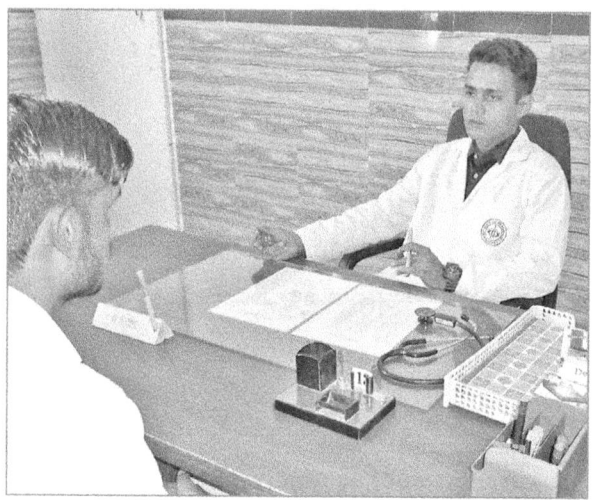

Fig. 5.2: Backward leaning: Wrong posture.

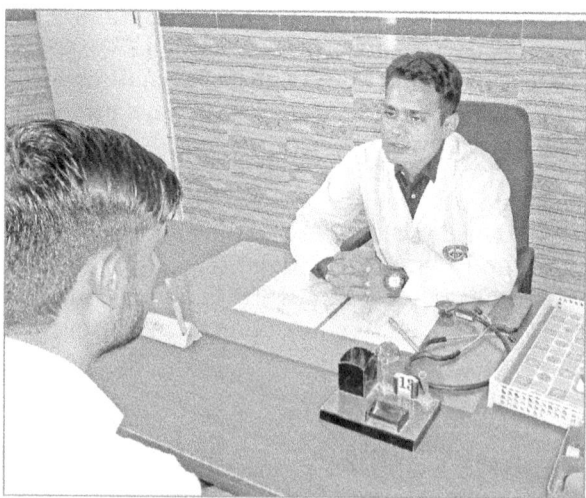

Fig. 5.3: Sprinter's position: Right posture.

Chapter 5: Elements of Communication

- Prefer to sit or stand in an open posture. Both arms should be free and open. Avoid closed postures, such as locking your arms in front of the chest or the groin region (fig leaf stance). Avoid locking your hands on your back region (stand-at-ease position) (**Figs. 5.4 to 5.6**).
- Do not keep your any of your hands in your pocket (**Fig. 5.7**).

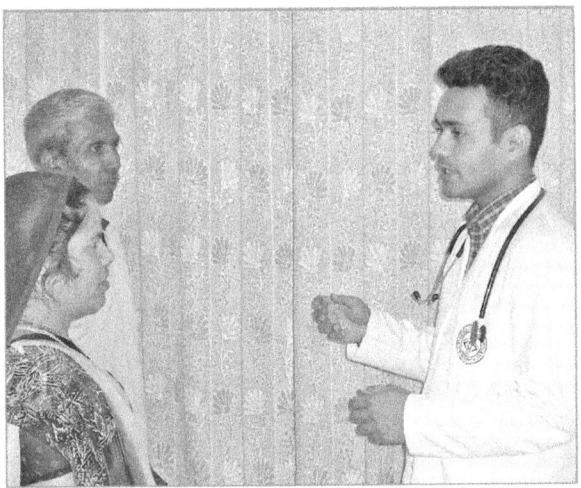

Fig. 5.4: Open posture.

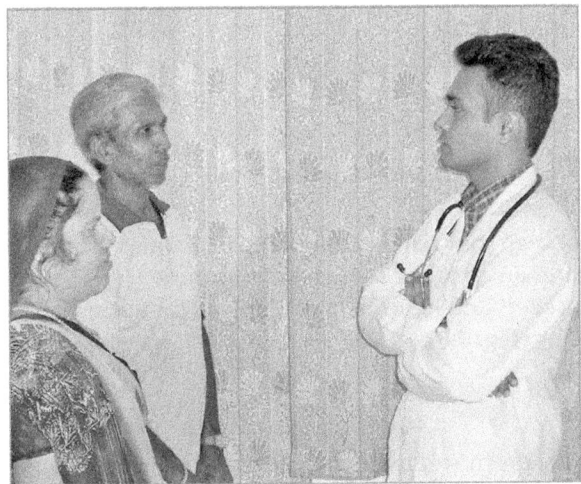

Fig. 5.5: Closed posture.

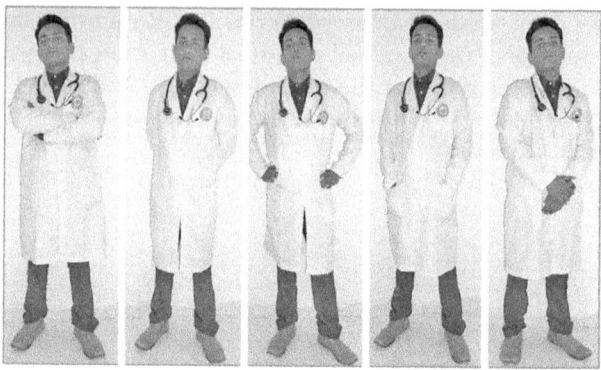

Fig. 5.6: Various types of wrong postures in standing position.

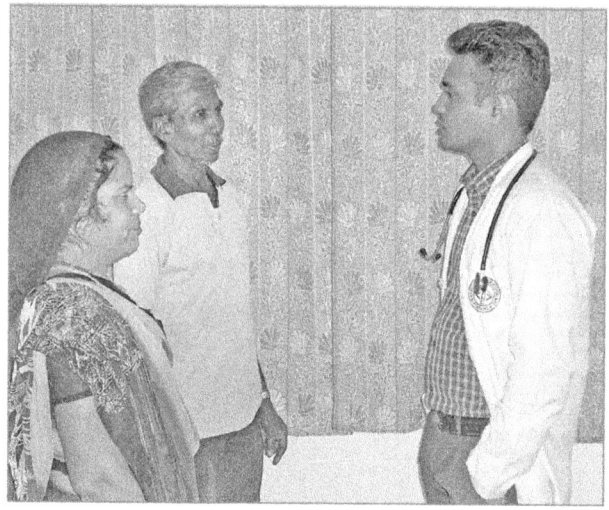

Fig. 5.7: Hands in pocket: Wrong posture.

- Do not keep your hands on your hip (arms akimbo position). This indicates an arrogant or aggressive attitude.
- Do not keep your hand on your chin and mouth, especially during speaking (**Fig. 5.8**).

Gesture

Gestures are the movements of some part (mainly hand and head) or whole of the body to express some idea or meaning. They are different from the sign language, which is used for communication with and

Chapter 5: Elements of Communication

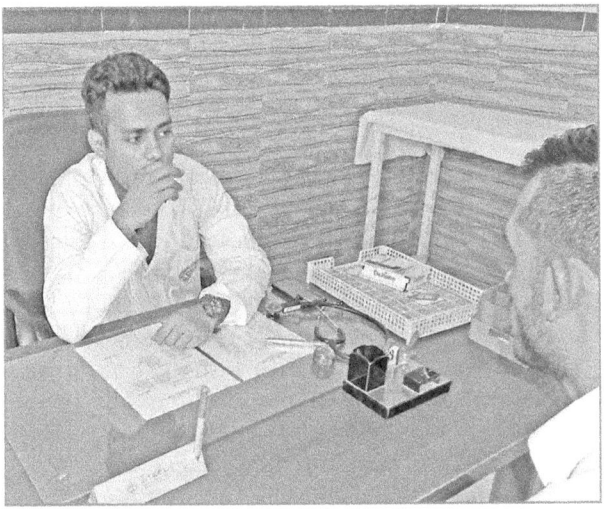

Fig. 5.8: Hand on mouth while speaking: Wrong position.

between deaf and dumb persons. A systematic study of the importance of gestures in communication is known as *kinesics*.

There are several ways to classify the commonly practiced gestures. One classification divides them in three groups:

Symbolic Gestures

These gestures are also known as emblems. These gestures are intentionally made by the person to convey some signal or message to another person. For example, waving the hand for *good bye*, showing the thumb for *good wishes*, crossed fingers for *good luck*, beckoning to *call* someone, up-down head nodding for *yes*, side-to-side head nodding for *no*, joining the palm of both hands for *namaste*, and many more.

These gestures can be made with/without speech. For example, while leaving someone, you can simply wave your hand or can say "bye-bye" along with the waving hand. In other words, they are made consciously or subconsciously, either to replace or to augment the effect of spoken words.

The meaning of some of these gestures may be different in different countries. For example, making a circle with your thumb and index finger is a sign of appreciation (OK) in many countries, but in Japan, it is considered as a sign for money and in Arabic countries, it is a sign of threat. Hence, one should be cautious while practicing such gestures at some alien place.

Conversational Gestures

These are the random movements of one or both hands which are subconsciously performed by the person only when he speaks (**Figs. 5.4 and 5.9**). They are also known as illustrators. These gestures differ from the symbolic gestures on following points:

- Symbolic gestures are mostly performed consciously while conversational gestures are subconscious movements.
- Symbolic gestures can be made with/without speech while conversational gestures are made only while the person is speaking (hence, they are called as conversational gestures). These movements start and stop with the speech only.
- Various types of symbolic gestures carry some specific meaning, which is decoded and understood by the receiver. In contrast, conversational gestures are random movements without any specific meaning.

Sometimes, these movements are performed subconsciously even when the other person is not in front of you, e.g., during telephonic conversation.

Different people have got different tendencies to perform these gestures. The overall effect of these movements is determined by

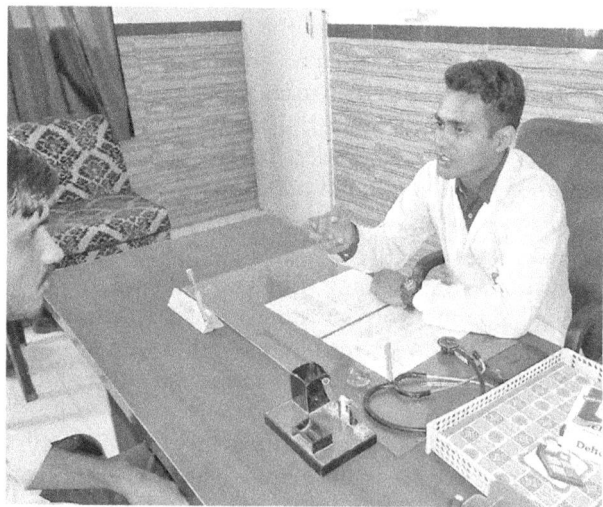

Fig. 5.9: Conversation gestures.

their various characters, such as frequency, speed, range, etc., of the hand movements.

The greatest advantage of proper use of conversational gestures is that they make the person look more confident in communication. This can be felt by watching the speech of some famous politicians and news readers.

This is another advantage of keeping an open posture during communication, as your hands are free to perform these gestures during your speech. In one interesting study, participants were divided in three groups and were asked to speak in different conditions. In first group, both arms of participants were immobilized. In second group, only one arm was kept free while both arms were kept free in the third group. It was found that the restriction of movements of hands led to decrease of fluency of speech and increase in difficulty to find the proper words.

Adapters

These are not the true gestures. These are frequent purposeless movements made by some persons during communication. Some common examples are leg shaking, foot shaking, head scratching, nail biting, adjusting the spectacles, clicking the pen, etc. (**Fig. 5.10**). They can be made on their own body part (self-focused, such as repeatedly

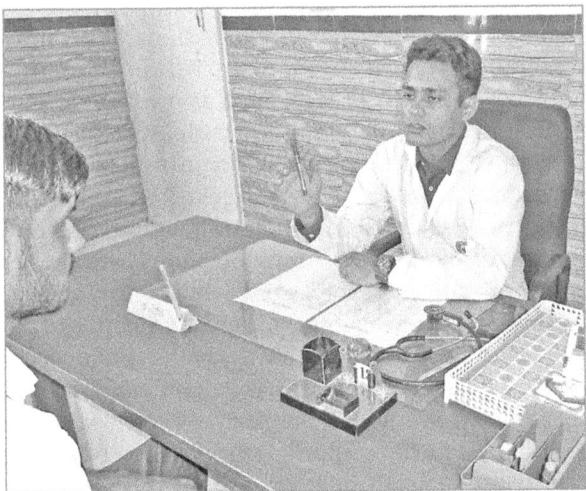

Fig. 5.10: Adapter: Fidgeting with pen.

touching the nose or curling the hair) or on some surrounding object (object focused, such as playing with the paper weight on table).

Some people are habitual of performing some specific movements frequently or continuously and subconsciously. In fact, these movements can be considered as strong distracters in communication, as they make the person look nervous (e.g., leg shaking) or disinterested (e.g., pen clicking, playing with some object) during conversation.

Most of the gestures mentioned above are made by various movements of hands (manual gestures). There are several other gestures which are made by some other body part (nonmanual gestures). Head nodding is the most important example of the nonmanual gesture. As the conversational gestures are made while person is speaking, head nodding is performed subconsciously while the person is listing to someone. Proper head movement during listening gives a positive feedback to the speaker and encourages him to speak more.

Like the conversational gesture, one should also be careful about various features of head nodding, such as speed, range, frequency, etc. For example, it is better to perform slow and lengthy nods, as rapid and small movements may make the person feel that you are in hurry. Similarly, intermittent head movements are better, as they look more natural than the continuous up and down movement of head.

Facial Expressions

Human face can make thousands of expressions, either intentionally or subconsciously. These are made by various combinations of movements of some parts of face, such as eyes, eyelids, eyebrows, lips, nose, and cheeks. Some common examples of the feelings which can be conveyed through some specific type of facial expressions are happiness, sadness, surprise, anger, disgust, fear, confusion, etc.

During face-to-face communication, these expressions are mostly made subconsciously. Communication is always better if the person has some specific expressions while speaking or listening. The expressions made during speaking greatly augment the impact of spoken message. For example, it is always better to convey some good news with happy facial expressions and some bad news with some degree of sadness on your face. Similarly, a person will always get a positive feedback if he finds appropriate variation of expressions on face of his listener, such as smile, amused, surprised, etc. (**Fig. 5.11**). No one will be encouraged to speak to a person who is listening to him with a mask-like expressionless face. Expressions of listener make the

Chapter 5: Elements of Communication

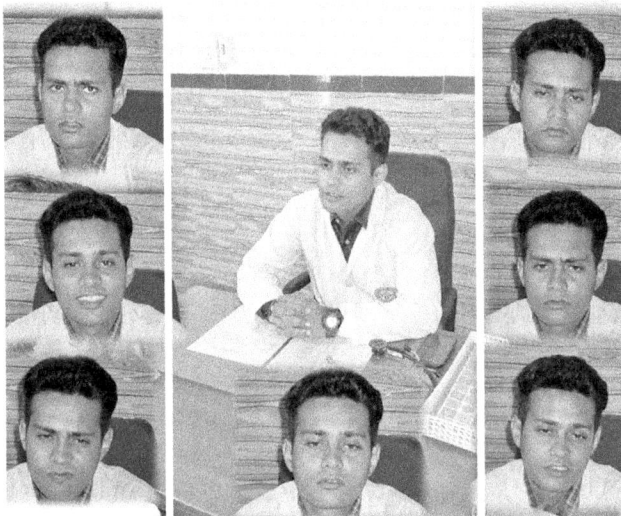

Fig. 5.11: Various types of facial expressions.

speaker feel that he is not just hearing the spoken words, but he is also understanding the conveyed message.

Eye Contact

It is the moment when two persons simultaneously look in each other's eyes during face-to-face conversation. It is also known as the mutual gaze. A systematic study of the role of this element in communication is known as *oculesics*.

During communication, it is important to be careful about various parameters of eye contact, such as duration, frequency and direction of eye movements, blink rate, etc. Proper eye contact makes the person look more confident during speaking (**Fig. 5.3**). Similarly, listening with a good eye contact makes you look attentive and interested in listening. In some studies, it is suggested that eye contact should be maintained for 70% of time during speaking and for 90% of time during listening. Total avoidance of eye contact makes you look under confident and disinterested in communication (**Fig. 5.12**). In contrast, continuous staring and infrequent blinking of the person can make the other one uncomfortable after sometime.

Like the other factors of nonverbal communication, the pattern of eye contact also varies from person to person. Some people avoid making eye contact during speaking or listening or both. This is known

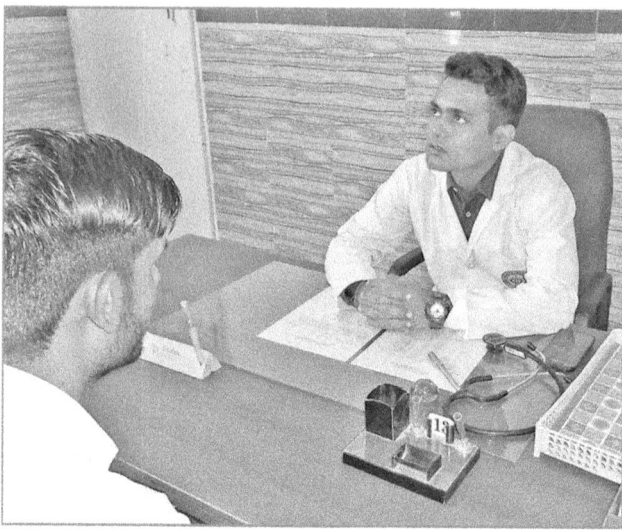

Fig. 5.12: Eye aversion: Poor eye contact during communication.

as eye aversion. Moreover, the pattern of eye contact of some people depends on seniority and gender of the other person, i.e., they find it difficult to make proper eye contact with the persons of opposite gender.

It is important to be careful about where to look during the breaks of eye contact. Human eyes differ from the eyes of other animals in the fact that a larger part of sclera (white) of human eyes is visible. Because of this, a person can accurately judge that you are looking at which part of his face or body. Sometimes, this can act as distracter in proper communication. For example, a young girl will certainly become uncomfortable if, during conversation, you start looking at some acne on her cheek. Similarly, if you look at mobile, wrist watch, or wall clock frequently, the person may feel that you are in hurry and not interested in communicating with him.

It is better to be careful and attentive toward our eye contact while talking to a small group of persons (such as patient with his relatives). During speaking, try to make intermittent eye contact with almost everyone in the group, depending upon their relative importance in communication. Eye contact is a sign of engagement. If you make eye contact with only one person, after sometime, the others may start feeling neglected.

Chapter 5: Elements of Communication

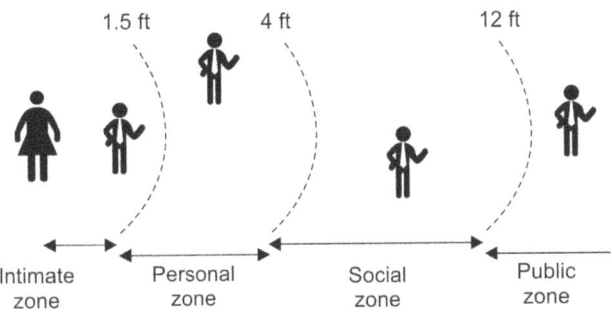

Fig. 5.13: Interpersonal distance zones.

Distance

The physical distance between two persons during communication is known as the interpersonal distance. It is important to keep this distance in mind during face-to-face conversation. A systematic study of role and impact of this distance during communication is known as *proxemics*.

In general, the distance of about 1.5 feet from a person is considered as the intimate distance and this zone around him is called as the intimate zone. The person will be comfortable only if some intimate person (such as spouse, parents, or any other family member) is standing in this zone (the range of this zone is shorter in some countries, where people prefer to stand very close to each other during conversation) (**Fig. 5.13**).

The area beyond this zone is known as personal zone, which extends from 1.5 to 4 feet. This zone is appropriate to stand or sit during face-to-face communication.

Hence, except for the time when physical contact is essential (e.g., during examination of a patient), one should always prefer to stay in personal zone and to not to encroach in the intimate zone of the person. At the same time, it is also wrong to stand far away from any person, as both may not be clearly audible to each other. Moreover, this may give the person a feeling of being neglected and ignored (e.g., a doctor talking to an admitted patient from the door of his room).

The intimate distance can be roughly imagined as equal to *one arm's length*. This precaution is even more important when someone is communicating with a person of opposite gender.

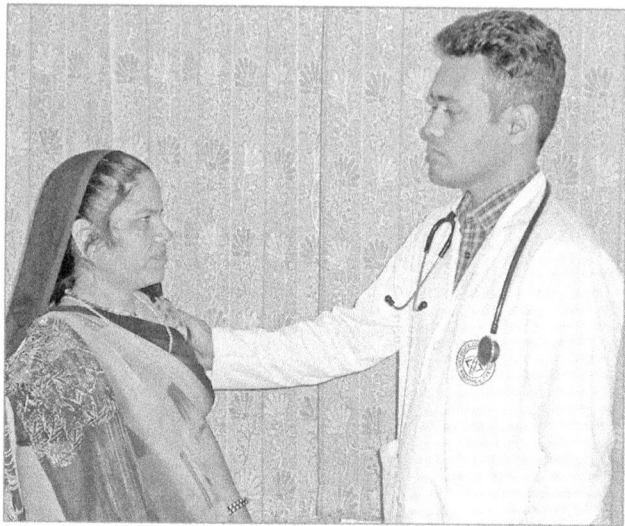

Fig. 5.14: Physical contact during communication.

Touching

There are several acts of physical contact between two persons during communication, such as hand shaking, hand on shoulder, pet on back, etc. Like the element of distance, the custom of these acts also varies in different countries. In some places, people prefer to make frequent physical contacts during communication while they are considered as unacceptable at some other place. The study of the role of physical contact during communication is known as *haptics*.

During communication, one should be careful about the impact of these acts. Apart from the culture of country, the age and gender of the persons play a very important role here. For example, while explaining about the prognosis of disease, it will be quite sympathetic and acceptable if young male doctor places his hand on the shoulder of an elderly male person, but the same act may not be acceptable if he does the same with a young female patient (**Fig. 5.14**).

How to Assess and Improve your Nonverbal Communication?

Following are some of the common and easy methods for a person to assess and improve his own nonverbal communication:

- *Self-awareness:* As described earlier, majority of our nonverbal communication is coded and decoded at subconscious level. Hence, a lot of self-assessment can be done by any person simply by focusing his mind on himself only. He can simply ask few questions to himself, such as *What do I do while talking to the others?, How do I stand?, Where do I keep my hand?, Do I make proper eye contact?, Do I nod my head while listening?,* and many more. This will help him in assessing his strength and weaknesses during communication.
- *Observation:* We meet and observe hundreds of people every day, in some or the other situation. A great amount of nonverbal communication can be learnt by watching the body language of people around us. Similarly, same practice can be done by observing the various elements of body language (such as gestures, expressions, etc.) of different people in movies, serials, interviews, news debates, etc. Volume of video should be turned off, as it will help you in concentrating only on the nonverbal communication of various characters.
- *Talking in front of a mirror:* By talking to himself in front of a mirror, a person can assess several elements of his body language like posture, gestures, and facial expressions. This method has been commonly practiced by various theater and movie artists, politicians, public speakers, etc. Unfortunately, this method is not useful for assessing the eye contact of the person as he will have to fix his gaze on his mirror image only.
- *Video recording:* This is probably the best and complete method of analysis of your body language. By watching the recorded video of your conversation with your friend, you can assess all three elements (verbal, paraverbal, and nonverbal) of communication. Moreover, this recording can also be preserved for comparison in future.

Section 3

Format of Medical History

Section Outline

- What, Why, and How to ask?
- Patient's Profile
- Presenting Complaints
- History of Presenting Complaints
- Past History
- Personal History
- Family History
- Menstrual and Obstetric History
- Drug History
- Allergy History
- Case History of Pediatric Patients

CHAPTER 6

What, Why, and How to ask?

There is only one rule for being a good talker—learn to listen.
—**Christopher Morley**

The process of history taking involves a series of specific questions which are asked by a doctor to the patient, mainly to make a provisional diagnosis of his disease. The art of history taking can be easily understood by keeping three questions in your mind: *"What to ask?", "Why to ask?"* and *"How to ask?"* These should be considered as the three essential pillars of art of history taking.

1. What to ask?

Out of the three questions, this is the simplest one to answer. Right from his student life, every doctor is trained with a specific *format* of history taking, which is available in all books on clinical examination.

There is no single, standard format which can be used for all types of patients in all over the world. For instance, there is a significant difference between format used for gynecological patients and that for psychiatric patients. While *menstrual and obstetric history* is stressed more for a gynecological patient, *personal history* will be a major section while interrogating a psychiatric patient.

Besides, there can also be some regional variation in importance of several questions. For example, the history of *tuberculosis* is quite important for a patient in India, but it is not of much importance for every patient in UK. Conversely, a physician can frankly ask about the *sexual history* to an adolescent girl in the Western world, but the same enquiry should be done more cautiously in our country.

2. Why to ask?

All the points mentioned in the format of history taking *are not equally important for all the patients*. For example, the history of alcohol consumption is more important for a patient presenting with cirrhosis of liver while history of diabetes is more significant for a patient with a nonhealing ulcer of foot. Hence, an enquiry of diabetes from a cirrhotic patient and of alcohol addiction from a patient with foot ulcer will not be of very much significance during clinical practice.

In other words, for any disease, all the questions of the standard format of history can be broadly divided in "very important", "important," and "unimportant" categories, from the point of view of their relative significance in diagnosis and management of the disease. For example, in case of a patient presenting with hematemesis, history of *addiction* (alcohol) will be very important, *dietary* history (spicy diet) will be important, but *residence, sleep, marital status*, etc., will be relatively unimportant questions to be asked. On the other hand, in case of a female presenting with a painless lump in her breast, enquiry of *family history* will be very important, her *menstrual and obstetric history* will be important while many other points, such as *religion, occupation, addiction,* etc., will be comparatively unimportant for making diagnosis and treatment plan her disease.

As a part of his medical training, every student is expected to ask all the questions to all the patients. Moreover as he is in early stage of learning, it is difficult for him to confidently decide the relative importance of various questions for various diseases. But at the same time, he should start learning about this type of segregation of questions in early stage. It would help him in categorizing the questions in his future life. It may be difficult for him initially, but gradually, with increasing theoretical and clinical knowledge, he will be able to select the relatively important questions for different diseases.

3. How to ask?

This is the most difficult but interesting task of history taking. It is all about learning *the best way* of asking a particular question to a particular patient. Students learn this skill subconsciously, mostly by observing the communication of their teachers or seniors with various types of patients. Most of the available literature on clinical aspects of different subjects has focused mainly on the "examination" part, while "history taking" is confined to the first few pages only.

No one can make a standard way by which all the questions can be asked to all types of patients. The appropriate method of asking a question to a patient depends on various factors such as age, gender, education, socioeconomic status, etc. For example, imagine that two patients have visited you with almost similar complaints. One is a 20-year-old female college student, and the other one is a 60-year-old illiterate man from a nearby village. Now, you will be having similar questions (What to ask?) and similar reasons (Why to ask?) for both of them. But still, you will ask several questions in different ways (How to ask?), as there will be a significant difference in their understanding and intellectual level. The art of history taking is mainly about the tailoring of questions according to the understanding of your patients.

This section is mainly focused on answering the same question—"*How to ask?*" It will guide the students and doctors to the most practical way of asking a particular question of medical history from the patients of different age, sex, and socioeconomic status. This knowledge will definitely improve their confidence while interacting with various types of patients, and that will lead to a more successful session of communication with the patient.

FORMAT OF MEDICAL HISTORY

Format of the medical history is a set of multiple questions arranged in a specific sequence, which are asked to a patient by a student or doctor.

It is desirable but difficult to make a format which includes all relevant questions for taking medical history of *all types* of patients. A format which is suitable for some common medical or surgical disease of an adult patient may not be suitable for taking history of pediatric or psychiatric patients. Because, some information, such as antenatal history, immunization, development history, etc., are more important in pediatric age groups, but they are not of much use for adult patients. Similarly, in contrast to other diseases, history of a psychiatric patient needs a special emphasis on his personal history and family history.

Moreover, some major to minor variations have been observed in the formats used in different books. The format which is used for description of history taking in this book is as follows:
1. Patient's Profile:
    - Name
    - Age
    - Sex
    - Residence
    - Religion
    - Occupation
    - Socioeconomic status

2. Presenting complaints
3. History of presenting complaints
4. Past history
   - History of any significant disease (such as tuberculosis, diabetes, hypertension, etc.)
   - History of hospitalization
   - History of any surgery
   - History of any other significant event
   - History of similar complaints in the past
5. Personal history
   - Sleep
   - Diet
   - Appetite
   - Weight change
   - Addiction
   - Bladder and bowel habits
   - Marital status and children
6. Family history
7. Obstetric and menstrual history
8. Drug history
9. Allergy history

CHAPTER 7

Patient's Profile

The art of communication is the language of leadership.
—*James Humes*

This is the first section of the standard format of medical history. It collects following general information from the patient:
1. Name
2. Age
3. Sex
4. Residence
5. Religion
6. Occupation
7. Socioeconomic status

NAME

General conversation with any new person mostly starts with asking his/her name. It is not uncommon to find two patients with the same name in the same ward of the hospital. So, to avoid any confusion, students should develop a habit of asking the complete name of the patient, i.e., along with father's/husband's name and surname.

Sometimes, because of certain social customs, many women hesitate in speaking out their husband's name. In such a case, name of her husband should be asked from any accompanying relative of the patient.

Frequent use of patient's name during conversation (e.g., Shyamlal ji, Geeta bai, Mr Rohit, Miss Shalini, etc.) will give him a feeling of caring attitude and personal attention from the doctor.

AGE

Age of the patient is the first information which can make a significant impact in presuming the diagnosis of disease. Two different diseases

can present with similar signs and symptoms in two different age groups. Following are few examples:
- *Benign prostatic hyperplasia* is a common cause of straining in micturition in elderly people, but if the same symptom is complained in a younger age group, the diagnosis goes more in favor of *urethral stricture*.
- Abdominal (renal) lump and hematuria are more likely to be because of *renal cell carcinoma* in a 35-year-old patient, but when the same features are seen in a 3-year-old child, *Wilms' tumor* would be the most probable diagnosis.
- Breast lump in an adolescent female is more likely to be *fibroadenoma,* but one should suspect *carcinoma* if the patient is middle aged or elderly.

In general, while congenital problems are more common in younger age groups, malignancies and degenerative disorders are commonly seen in elderly patients.

So, it is important in medical history to know about the age of every patient. But sometimes, it may not be easy for some patients to tell their accurate age to a student or doctor. They frankly accept that they do not have any idea of their age because of their illiteracy or poverty. Such a strange reply may be quite surprising for young student and he may even feel annoyed on this careless attitude of the patient. This is a common obstacle faced during communication with elderly and illiterate patients. This happens because patients think that the student wants to know about their *exact age* and they may not be aware of it. Hence, whenever you get such a reply from any patient, give him the liberty to tell his *approximate age* at least. Now, he may respond in some range, such as 40–45 years, 60–70 years, etc. This answer is quite sufficient to get an idea about his approximate age. Proceed ahead by selecting a single figure from this range, without wasting any time in finding his accurate age.

Still, some other patients are unable to quote even their approximate age. In such cases, some indirect methods can be used to reach to some conclusion. Following are few examples:
- An adolescent female and her parents were unable to give any answer about her age. It was found that she had attained menarche 3 years back. On this basis, the doctor presumed her to be around 14-year-old.
- An elderly female did not remember her age, but she had attained menopause 5 years back. Her approximate age was considered to be about 50 years.

- An adult female was married since 4 years. On this basis, she was presumed to be of about 22 years of age.
- A middle-aged rural man could only inform that his elder most child (daughter) was married last year. On this basis, he was calculated to be approximately 40-year-old.
- Parents of a child were not sure about his exact age or date of birth. He was found to be a student of 3rd standard and so, was presumed to be around 8-year-old.

These indirect methods will help the students in saving their precious time during history taking and will lead to a smooth and confident communication with such patients.

SEX

Out of all the information, this is the most obvious one and there is no need to ask about it, except for newborns and infants. Personally, I prefer to call it as *gender*, especially while conversing with the students in front of the patients, as the word *sex* has got a dual meaning.

It is quite obvious that the diseases related to external and internal genital organs will be exclusively found in the patients of that gender only. Still, there are some diseases of other organs which are more commonly seen in patients of a particular gender. For example, thyroid and gallbladder diseases are more common in females. Similarly, some diseases, such as inguinal hernia, carcinoma stomach, and carcinoma lung are more commonly seen in male patients.

RESIDENCE

Some diseases are more prevalent in a particular geographical location. The information of residence of patients may provide a strong clue in favor of their diagnosis. Following are few well-known examples:
- *Goiter* is more commonly seen in people living in Himalayan regions.
- *Filariasis* is more prevalent in Bihar and Orissa states.
- *Carcinoma stomach* is more common in Japan.

There are many more examples supporting the importance of residence in diagnosis of disease. But practically, it is more important for a doctor to know about different *areas of city or district* where he is practicing. For example, if he finds that a child with abdominal pain resides in some slum area of his city, he will start thinking more about diseases, such as worm infestation or gastroenteritis. Infectious diseases (such as tuberculosis, scabies, worm infestation, etc.) are relatively uncommon in people living in posh areas of town. Similarly, patients with respiratory diseases are more likely to have some industrial etiology if they belong to the industrial areas of their city. With experience, a doctor may notice higher prevalence of some diseases (e.g., renal stones) in some zones of districts around him. In such cases, the information of patient's residence will help him presuming the diagnoses in future.

It is often advised to the students to record complete postal address of the patient. But sometimes, it may be difficult to ask and record it in some cases, especially of rural patients (as their postal address may not be as simple and straightforward as of the urban patients). Moreover, complete postal address is essential only for follow-up of the patients after discharge and an undergraduate medical student has hardly got any role in it. So, during history taking, it is easy and sufficient to ask only about the name of *village* and *district* of rural patients.

RELIGION

Some diseases are more prevalent in people of a particular religion or caste. For example, in our country, thalassemia is commonly seen in people of *Sindhi* and *Punjabi* caste while sickle cell anemia is more common in *Rajput* caste. In contrast, some diseases are comparatively less common in some communities, e.g., carcinoma penis is rare in *Jews* and *Muslims* due to the practice of religious circumcision.

There are four major religions in our country (Hindu, Muslim, Sikh, and Christians) which are divided in multiple castes and subcastes. Relative population of different religions varies from place to place.

Religion of some patients is obvious from their name and appearance (e.g., Muslim, Sikh, etc.). In such cases, there is no need to ask about it separately.

In most of the diseases, it is easy and sufficient to note about the religion only. Information about the caste of the patient is needed only in selected cases. Most of the students know only the major religions and some of the common castes. In many cases, caste of the patient may be some new and unknown word for the students, especially from the patients of rural and tribal areas.

Some castes are obvious from *surname* of the patient, e.g., *Manjrekar* for Marathi caste, *Wadhwani* for Sindhi caste, etc. Still a confirmation should be made by asking the patient, as it is not uncommon to find people with same surname belonging to different castes. For example, *Shah* surname is common in Gujarati, Jain, and Muslim people while *Bhatia* is a common surname in both Sindhi and Punjabi castes.

OCCUPATION

Some of the diseases are strongly related to people involved with a particular type of occupation. Following are some well-known examples:
- Varicose veins commonly develop in people who stand for prolonged period during their jobs, e.g., traffic constables, bus conductors, etc.
- Carcinoma bladder is more common in workers of industries, such as rubber, textiles, petrochemicals, etc.
- Implantation dermoid is commonly seen in people who frequently suffer from prick injury during their work, e.g., tailors, gardeners, etc.
- Some pulmonary diseases are intimately associated with particular occupation, such as silicosis (in miners), asbestosis (in asbestos workers), coal workers' pneumoconiosis (in coal miners), byssinosis (in textile workers), etc.
- Hepatitis B is commonly seen in person exposed to the blood of infected individuals, e.g., in healthcare professionals, such as doctors, nurses, etc.
- Radiology technicians are at higher risk of developing some malignancies (such as leukemia, thyroid cancer, etc.) due to chronic exposure of ionizing radiations.

In general, occupation of a person increases the risk of some diseases by bringing a chronic change in his lifestyle or by exposing him to certain chemicals, injuries, etc. So, in such cases, this information provides a strong clue for diagnosis of the disease.

Most of the patients visiting to a medical college hospital belong to low socioeconomic class. Many of them are *laborers* by occupation and so, this is the most common answer received by the students while taking history in medical college. But, this word is of no significance in making any diagnosis as it does not tell anyone about the *type of work* done by the patient. For example, all the people who work in fields, factories, road construction, building construction, etc., will call themselves as laborer, but all of them are exposed to different types of chemicals and injuries. A field laborer is more exposed to soil, crops, insect and animal bites, etc., while another laborer who is working for road construction will have different exposures, such as heat, coal tar, etc. In contrast, a laborer in some factory will get more exposure of various chemicals used at his working place. So, wherever any patient calls himself a laborer, it is essential to ask about the place where he works and the type of work done by him.

In some cases, it is more important to know about the lifestyle of patient during his working hours. For example:

> A middle-aged person presented with complaints of pain and swelling in both lower limbs since few weeks. On asking about the occupation, he informed that he owned a medical store. On further enquiry, it was found that for most of the time in a day, he was working in standing position in his medical store. This information guided the doctor to suspect *varicose veins* in his case. Clinical examination and investigations supported and confirmed this suspicion.

> A young man presented with complaints of headache and blurring of vision. On asking about his occupation, he informed that he was an employee at a garment showroom. But on asking about his lifestyle, he revealed that he was working in billing section of the showroom and so, a major part of his day was spent in front of computer screen.

> A 29-year-old male, who was an employee in a multinational company, presented with complaint of burning pain in epigastric region since 1 month. He was nonsmoker, nonalcoholic, and consumed nonspicy food. The physician was able to make a provisional diagnosis of *peptic ulcer* on basis of his stressful lifestyle (long working hours, inadequate sleep, irregular meals, pressure of achieving targets, etc.).

In some cases, it is important to know also about the duration since the patient is involved with his occupation. Most of the occupational diseases (such as malignancies) develop only after chronic exposure to harmful substances. So, the information about occupation becomes even more significant if patient is involved in it since a long duration.

It is not necessary that all patients are essentially involved with some occupation. So, when someone asks any patient about *what does he do*, it is not uncommon to get answers, such as housewife, student, retired, unemployed, etc. A patient should not be called as *unemployed*, if he is not involved with any occupation since few days or weeks. In most of the cases, it is the disease of the patient which makes him unable to perform his regular job. So, whenever, it is found that patient is not doing anything since sometime, he should be asked about the type of work he used to do in earlier days.

SOCIOECONOMIC STATUS

Some diseases are more commonly seen in people of low socioeconomic status (e.g., tuberculosis, scabies, etc.) while others are more prevalent in high-class families (e.g., diabetes, hypertension, etc.).

Many classification systems are available to estimate the socioeconomic class of the patient, but the most commonly used in our country is the "Kuppuswamy's Socioeconomic Status Scale". It is based on three parameters (education, occupation, and family income) and stratifies the population in five socioeconomic classes (upper, upper middle, lower middle, upper lower, and lower classes).

Methodical estimation of exact socioeconomic class is difficult and mostly unnecessary from the point of view of routine medical history. For practical purpose, patients can be simply divided in three basic groups (upper, middle, and lower). Most of the patients in government and medical college hospitals belong to low socioeconomic class. Additionally, it can be presumed from their appearance also. But still, a superficial enquiry about education and income of patients should be done as occasionally, appearance of some patients may not match with their socioeconomic class.

Out of these two parameters (education and income), it is comparatively easier to know about the education of the patients. Most of the patients from low socioeconomic class are either illiterate or educated up to certain levels of school only.

Proper method of asking about the income of the patient largely depends on the type of his occupation. Most of the laborers are comfortable in informing about their daily wages and so, should be asked accordingly. In contrast, an employee of some government or private field (such as clerk, peon, watchman, etc.) will be able to mention his income in figures of his monthly salary. On the other hand, farmers are mostly comfortable in quoting their annual income from their fields. So, the question about his income should be modified according to the occupation of the patient.

CHAPTER 8

Presenting Complaints

Symptoms, then are in reality nothing but the cry from suffering organs.
—*Jean-Martin Charcot*

This section is also known as the section of "chief complaints". It is the most important of all sections of format of history taking as it enquires about the problem which has brought the patient to the doctor. In clinical practice, doctors mostly start their conversation with patients with this section only.

THE MEANING OF PRESENTING COMPLAINTS

As the name suggests, this section mainly focuses on the complaints with which any patient is *presenting* to the doctor. In other words, the patient may be having several chronic complaints of variable severity. But, the major attention should be paid to the complaints which have brought him to the hospital at present. For example, an elderly patient presents in surgical OPD with a complaint of nonhealing ulcer on his left foot for 2 months. He is diabetic for 4 years and is suffering from constipation for 10 years. Also, he is having a swelling behind his right pinna since the age of 15 years. In his case, only nonhealing ulcer should be considered as the *presenting complaint* as presently, he has come here only for the treatment of his foot ulcer. All other diseases should be mentioned in other suitable sections of the format, e.g., past history, personal history, etc.

Single Disease: Multiple Symptoms

Many diseases lead to several symptoms of variable severity (e.g., acute appendicitis cause abdominal pain, fever, vomiting, etc.). Sometimes, when patient is asked about his presenting complaints, he mentions only about the *most severe* symptom and forgets to inform about other

Chapter 8: Presenting Complaints

problems, especially if they are mild in intensity and/or occasional in frequency. So, never presume by his single answer that the he is suffering from only one complaint. Instead, you should always confirm or exclude the presence of any other symptoms by asking the patient as: *"Kya aapko aur bhi kuchh takleef hai?"* (Do you have any other complaints?). For example:

> A 40-year-old male patient with renal cell carcinoma visited to a surgical clinic. Initially, he complained only about dull pain in his left loin since few months. But when the surgeon asked him about *any other complaint*, he informed him about additional complaints of some episodes of hematuria and a painless swelling in his left scrotum (varicocele).

Whether informed by the patient or extracted by the physician, the second complaint plays an important role in making a provisional diagnosis in many cases. For example, if a patient presents with the chief complaint of *fever*, the second complaint will guide the physician toward specific systems, as:
- *If associated with cough and expectoration:* Possibility of respiratory infection
- *If associated with burning in micturition:* Possibility of urinary infection
- *If associated with diarrhea:* Possibility of gastrointestinal infection
- *If associated with jaundice:* Possibility of hepatobiliary disease, complicated malaria, etc.
- *If associated with tender swelling at some part of the body:* Possibility of cellulitis or abscess
- *If associated with altered sensorium or unconsciousness:* Possibility of CNS infections, such as meningitis, cerebral malaria, etc.

For this purpose, only open-ended questions should be used for asking about additional symptoms (e.g., "Do you have any other complaint?"). Closed questions should be avoided, especially in early phases of conversation (e.g., "Do you feel like vomiting?' or "Do you feel some distension of your abdomen?"). The difference between open-ended and closed question has been explained in next chapter.

Following are few reasons for why some patients do not inform about *all* of their complaints in first instance:
- Complaints which are of comparatively *less severity* are usually forgotten by the patient who is having some severe problem.

For example, a patient of ureteric stone with sever colicky pain may forget to mention about the complaints of mild fever and burning in micturition.
- Patient with some chronic disease may forget to mention about the complaints which have occurred only *occasionally* in long course of their disease. For example, a patient with chronic constipation forgot to inform about the episode of rectal bleeding, which had occurred around 2 months back.
- Some patients may not be aware of importance of some symptoms in relation to their disease. For example, a patient with swelling in neck may not feel it significant to tell the surgeon about additional complaint of diarrhea. It is major information if some thyroid pathology is suspected.

So, it should be remembered that it is a natural tendency of many patients to inform only about the major and most troublesome problem in the first instance. Maximum possible attempt should be made to enquire about additional symptoms, if any, before finalizing the list of chief complaints. A single disease can give rise to multiple symptoms and it is essential to know about all of them to make a proper provisional diagnosis.

Moreover, sometimes, it is essential to know about all the symptoms of the patient to plan the management. For example, benign prostatic hyperplasia is a common disease of old age which presents with a combination of wide variety of symptoms, such as increased frequency, urgency, poor stream, dribbling, etc. If an elderly patient presents with the only complaint of increased frequency of micturition, it is essential for the doctor to confirm about the presence or absence of other commonly associated symptoms. This will help him in deciding the severity of disease and to plan further management accordingly.

Occasionally, when asked about any additional symptom, some patient may inform about some complaint which cannot be correlated with his present disease. For example, an elderly patient presented with complaint of pain in his left lower limb for 1 month. When he was asked about *any other* complaint, he informed about a swelling over his back for 1 year. Now, despite of being a symptom, this swelling (which is probably a *sebaceous cyst*) cannot be correlated with chief complaint of this case (of limb pain). Moreover, it was present since a long time before the onset of his presenting complaint. Sometimes, it may become difficult for a medical student to decide the importance of such additional complaints with presenting illness of patient. But still, whenever in doubt, he should *include* such additional complaints in his presentation.

Chapter 8: Presenting Complaints

Unusual Answers

Sometimes, when asked about the complaints, instead of replying in simple and straightforward words (such as pain, vomiting, swelling, ulcer, etc.), some patient respond in some unusual ways. Following are few examples:

- Instead of speaking anything about the problem, the patient may simply *show* his complaint to the doctor. For example, if a patient is suffering from swelling of his right thumb, he will prefer to show his swollen thumb to the doctor instead of speaking anything about it.

    This commonly happens with surgical and dermatological problems (such as swelling, ulcer, pigmentation, rashes, etc.) which are present on exposed or exposable parts of the body (such as face, scalp, hand, forearm, etc.). Most of the times, this demonstration is sufficient as one can easily observe and understand the problem. So, instead of asking the patient to mention such lesions in some words, the student should proceed ahead with asking about other information related to it (such as duration, progression, etc.).

- Instead of telling some symptom, some patient may surprise you by telling the *diagnosis* of disease. For example, a patient with scrotal swelling tells about his problem as— *"Hernia ki takleef hai."* (I am suffering from *hernia*). Another patient with complaint of bleeding per rectum informs the doctor about it as— *"Mujhe bavaseer ho gayi hai."* (I am suffering from *piles*).

Many patients and their relatives have some common *misconceptions* about some diseases, mostly seen with poor and illiterate patients. For example:
  - Any scrotal or inguinoscrotal swelling (e.g., hernia, hydrocele, testicular tumor, varicocele, etc.) is called as a *hernia* by some patients.
  - Rectal bleeding due to any cause (e.g., hemorrhoids, fissure, carcinoma rectum, etc.) is called as *piles* by many people.
  - Appendicitis is a commonly known cause of acute abdomen. So, abdominal pain due to any cause may be called as *appendix* (lay term for appendicitis) by many people.
  - Abdominal pain which is associated with burning in micturition is complained as *pathari* (stone) by some patients.
  - Pneumonia is a well known term in general population, even to the illiterate persons. If a child is suffering from respiratory distress due to any cause (such as pneumonia,

viral bronchiolitis, asthma, etc.), his parents may present his complaint as of *pneumonia*.
- Symptoms, such as restlessness, headache, palpitation, etc., are complained as of *high BP* by some patients.
- Similarly, symptoms of fatigue and weakness are commonly complained as of *low BP* by some patients.
- A history of fever with chills may be complained as of *malaria* by some patients.

These all are common and well known diseases. They are so intimately associated with these symptoms that the people start thinking them synonymous to each other. So, instead of telling symptoms of disease, sometimes they directly tell the diagnosis of disease.

But, it is not necessary that the diagnosis complained by the patient is always the actual disease. There are many other causes of scrotal swelling (e.g., varicocele, testicular tumor, etc.) or rectal bleeding (e.g., carcinoma rectum), but all are called as *hernia* or *piles*, respectively, by such patients.

In some other cases, patient tells the diagnosis of disease simply because *he is aware of it*. The source of this knowledge may be some other doctor or the investigation reports. For example:

> Before visiting the surgical OPD, a patient with scrotal swelling had consulted some local doctor of his village. After his examination, he informed him that he was suffering from *hernia* and referred him to a higher center for its treatment. In OPD, when the intern asked him about his complaint, he confidently mentioned it as—"I am suffering from hernia". Accuracy of this diagnosis largely depends upon the knowledge and experience of first doctor and should never be accepted without confirming by proper history and examination.

> A patient visited his family physician with complaint of abdominal pain. After his examination, he advised him some investigations including abdominal sonography, which reported a stone of 15 mm size in his left kidney. After reading his report, patient directly visited to a surgeon and mentioned him his complaint as – "I have got a stone in my kidney."

Whatever, the reason may be, this type of response is quite common in clinical practice and should be dealt in a proper way, especially by young medical students. Here, though the words, such as *high BP, hernia, pneumonia,* etc., are spoken by the patients, still they cannot be accepted as the symptoms (as they are the signs and diagnoses). It will be incorrect and ridiculous if some student presents history of such patient as *"My patient is complaining of hernia since one year."*

A student should respond wisely in such cases. He should not react with surprise or disagreement to the belief of the patient, both verbally as well as nonverbally. Also, he should not make any attempt to find, that why, his patient thinks that he is suffering from *hernia* or *piles*. No attempt should be made to argue with the patient to correct his belief. Instead of it, student should calmly accept the spoken words and should ask the patient about the *trouble* caused by his disease.

Following short conversation between a student and a patient is an example of this method:

Student: *Aapko kya takleef hai?* (What is your complaint?)

Patient: *Bavaseer ki takleef hai.* (I am suffering from piles)

Student: *Kab se?* (Since how long?)

Patient: *Do mahine se.* (For two months.)

Student: *Theek. Aapke bavaseer se aapko kya takleef hoti hai?* (OK. What is the problem caused by your plies?)

Patient: *Tatti karne ke baad khoon aata hai.* (They bleed after passing stools.)

Student: *Theek. Aur kuchh takleef?* (OK. Any other complaint?)

Patient: *Kabhi kabhi bahar bhi aa jaate hai.* (Sometimes they even prolapse out.)

Now, it would be more logical and acceptable if you present the complaints of this patient in the form of some symptoms (such as rectal bleeding, mass prolapse after defecation, etc.), instead of presenting as *complaint of piles.*

Similarly, if some patient complains of high or low BP, student should calmly ask him to inform about the problems caused by his altered blood pressure, instead of presenting it as his presenting complaint.

- Sometimes, when asked about their complaints, instead of replying in terms of individual symptoms (such as pain, fever, etc.), some patients start describing the *details of the disease* since beginning. They start telling it like a story which includes the random features, such as onset of problem, characters of various symptoms, previous treatment, etc. All of these features are required for next section (History of presenting complaints) and this section needs only chief complaints with duration.

This may puzzle some inexperienced student as it is always easier for him to understand and record the complaints if they are presented by the patient in systematic and point wise manner. But, a student should remember that the *patients are not aware of the standard format of medical history*. So, he should not expect a *"one question-one answer"* type of conversation with each and every patient. In such cases, he should listen to his story carefully and simultaneously, he should pick up various symptoms with their duration. Finally, he should confirm about them by telling the list of various symptoms (with duration) to the patient and then should note them in chronological order. This method of extracting out the symptoms from a story can be learnt only by interacting more frequently with such type of patients. Following example is demonstrating the use of this method:

Student: Please tell me about your problem.

Patient: Sir, I was absolutely fine till 1 month back. Then I developed this complaint of abdominal pain, which becomes worse whenever I eat anything. It is even more sever whenever I eat some spicy food. I took some medicines from a doctor in my village, but it did not work. Instead of improving, I got another problem of vomiting for last 6–7 days.

Student (After listening everything carefully): So, you have got complaints of abdominal pain since a month and vomiting since a week. Right?

Patient: Yes, sir.

Student: Any other complaint?

Patient: No, sir.

After noting down these two symptoms as "presenting complaints", he proceeded for enquiring about their details for the section of "history of presenting complaints".

Duration of Complaints

It is difficult to make a provisional diagnosis of any disease exclusively on the basis of symptoms unless an enquiry is made about their *duration* also. Two diseases can present with almost similar symptoms but from different durations. Following are few well known examples to support the significance of duration of complaints in making the provisional diagnosis:

- Severe pain in lower limb since few hours favors the diagnosis of *embolism* while a pain since few weeks or months points toward some chronic peripheral vascular disease such as *atherosclerosis* or *Buerger's disease*.
- Cough and fever since few days is more likely to be because of *acute bronchitis* while same complaints since few weeks can be because of some chronic respiratory disease such as *tuberculosis*.
- A swelling which has developed and progressed in few days is more likely because of some *inflammatory* condition (e.g., abscess), while another swelling which is present since few months is more likely to be because of some *neoplastic* disease (benign or malignant).

In some cases, chronological sequence of occurrence of various symptoms affects the provisional diagnosis. For example:
- In cases of *inflammatory* diseases, pain occurs before appearance of swelling. On the other hand, in *neoplastic* diseases, a lump or swelling is noticed much before onset of pain.
- For a patient presenting with complaints of fever and headache, if the fever had started before the headache, *meningitis* is the probable cause. But if the headache had started before the fever, it is likely to be a case of *subarachnoid hemorrhage*.

So, it is essential to know about the duration of various complaints which can be in terms of hours, days, weeks, months or years.

However, it may not always be possible for every patient to tell you the exact duration of his complaints. Sometimes, some patients give a vague and nonspecific reply of -*"since a long time"*, especially for the chronic complaints. This happens even more commonly in cases of elderly patients with poor memory. This should not bring the student any annoyance or surprise during conversation. Immediately, he should help the patient by giving him a liberty to tell about the *approximate* duration of his complaint as it is not essential to find out *exact* duration of symptoms in most of the cases. This method works for most of the patients and they come out with some better answer like 6–7 months or 4–5 years.

Occasionally, even this method fails to get any information and patient is unable to mention even about approximate duration of his complaints. In such cases, the student should first help him by asking that whether his problem is since few weeks or months or years. Then he should ask him to correlate the onset of symptoms with some *season* (such as summer, winter, etc.) or some major *event* (e.g., festival). For example:

Section 3: Format of Medical History

> A patient with complaint of abdominal pain presented to the doctor in August. He was unable to recall the duration of his complaints. He could only inform that it was since *few months*. Now, the doctor asked him to correlate the onset of his problem with some festival such as *Holi* or *Diwali*. He informed that he was alright during last *Diwali* but his problem had started just after the festival of *Holi*. On this basis, it was presumed that he was suffering from abdominal pain for 5 months.

Most of the patients from rural areas are intimately associated with agricultural practice. Sowing (*buvai*) and reaping (*kataai*) of major crops are the important events of their lives which can be correlated to know about the time of onset of their disease. For example, sowing and reaping of *soybean* is done in June and October, respectively. Similarly, *wheat* is sown in November and reaped in the month of March.

So, one can get an approximate idea of duration of disease by asking questions like *"Do you remember what was happening in fields when your disease started?"* or *"Were you alright during last winter?"* etc. This method can also be used to know about approximate time when some important events had occurred in the course of disease (e.g., hospitalization, surgery, any episode of aggravation of symptoms, etc.).

Some rural patients may not be able to mention the onset of disease or some major event in terms of Gregorian calendar (January, February, etc.), but they reply in the form of months of Hindu calendar (*Chaitra, Vaishakh,* etc.). So, the students are advised to have knowledge of different months of this calendar, and their relation with the months of Gregorian calendar **(Table 8.1)**.

TABLE 8.1: 12 months of Hindu calendar.

No.	Hindu calendar	Gregorian calendar
1.	Chaitra	March/April
2.	Vaishakh	April/May
3.	Jyeshtha	May/June
4.	Aashaad	June/July
5.	Shravan	July/August
6.	Bhadra	August/September
7.	Ashvin	September/October
8.	Kartik	October/November
9.	Agahaan	November/December
10.	Paush	December/January
11.	Maagh	January/February
12.	Falgun	February/March

Some patients correlate some specific event (such as onset of pain, last menstrual period, etc.) with *Amavasya* (dark moon night) or *Poornima* (full moon night) of Hindu calendar.

It is not uncommon to find a patient who *changes* the duration of his disease during conversation with the doctor. This usually happens in the cases where there is some *change in the severity* of disease. For example:

> A patient informed the student that he was suffering from abdominal pain since a week. Student noted down the complaint and duration, and started thinking about the probable differential diagnoses. But, during subsequent conversation, patient revealed the information that actually he was suffering from mild abdominal pain for 2 months, which had increased in severity since a week.

So, whenever the patient informs about the duration of his complaint, it is better to confirm it by asking that whether he was absolutely alright before that duration (*"Kya aap us ke pehle bilkul theek the?"*). Many a times, patients change the duration of their disease after getting this question. Maximum possible attempt should be made to confirm about the exact duration of disease before proceeding ahead.

How to Present the Symptoms?

A single disease can give rise to multiple symptoms. Following rules should be considered by the students while noting and presenting the list of chief symptoms of the patient:

1. *Chronological order:* It is never a rule that all symptoms of any disease should always start simultaneously. If a patient is presenting with more than one symptom, they should be recorded and presented in chronological order, i.e., what happened first should be placed on top of the list. It is not necessary that chronological order always matches with severity of disease. For example, a patient presented with complaint of severe abdominal pain for 2 days. On enquiring about any other complaint, he told that he was also suffering from mild fever since a week. Though his fever is less severe than the pain, still it should be mentioned on top of the list. i.e.,
   - Fever since 7 days
   - Abdominal pain since 2 days

2. *Order of severity:* If two complaints are occurring since same time, they should be arranged according to the order of severity. For example, if a patient complains of *severe* headache with *low grade* fever for 3 days, headache should get the priority in the list on the basis of its severity.

   It may not be always easy to stratify the complaints on the basis of severity. If multiple symptoms of same severity are occurring since same duration, the symptom which was complained *first* by the patient can be roughly considered as the more severe one.

   If two symptoms of the patient are occurring since same time, they should be mentioned individually and not together in a single sentence. For example, symptoms of the above-mentioned case should not be presented as—*"My patient is complaining of headache and fever for 3 days."*
   It would be better to present all the symptoms individually as:
   - Headache since 3 days
   - Fever since 3 days
3. *Special cases:*
   - If some diseases is progressively involving different parts or systems of the body, occurrence of every new event should be mentioned separately. For example, if a patient of Buerger's disease complains of pain in his left leg for 8 months and in right leg for 2 months, the complaints should be presented as:
     + Pain in left lower limb since 8 months
     + Pain in right lower limb since 2 months
   - If some patient presents with acute exacerbation (aggravation) of some chronic disease, both event should be mentioned separately. For example, if some cardiac patient says that he was having complaint of dyspnea on exertion for 2 years, but for 4 days, he is feeling dyspneic even in resting condition. His complaints should be presented as:
     + Difficulty in breathing on exertion since 2 years
     + Difficulty in breathing at rest since 4 days

Description of any *character* of symptoms should be avoided in section of presenting complaints, e.g., *high-grade* fever, *severe* headache, *colicky* abdominal pain, *nonbilious* vomiting, etc. These features should be described in next section (history of presenting complaints), and only major symptoms and their duration should be mentioned in the section of presenting complaints.

CHAPTER 9

History of Presenting Complaints

The doctor may also learn more about the illness from the way the patient tells the story than from the story itself.
—*James B Herrick*

This section is also known as "history of present illness (HPI)". It is the most important section of any medical history, as it includes a brief description of patient's disease right from its onset till present time. In this section, patient is enquired about following important information related to his disease:
- Onset of the disease
- Course (progression or regression) of the disease
- Characteristic features of major symptoms
- Treatment history
- Negative history

Onset of the Disease

The beginning of most of the diseases is usually spontaneous, but in some cases, there may be some significant event (e.g., trauma, insect bite, injection, medication, exertion, etc.) which has led to the onset of the disease. This information may provide a significant clue to the diagnosis. For example:

> A young male presented with severe pain in his right testicle since few hours. He revealed a history of sudden lifting of heavy weight in gymnasium. This information helped the physician in suspecting a diagnosis of testicular torsion.

> A child was brought with complaints of high-grade fever and a painful swelling on his buttock since few days. Parents revealed the history of injection of some medicine by a local doctor at the same site, 2 days before the onset of the swelling. On this basis, it was diagnosed as a case of post-injection abscess.

So, if any such event is found in the history of the patient, an attempt should be made to obtain the maximum possible details and it should be mentioned specifically during presentation.

But, if there is a significant time gap between the event and the onset of the disease, it would be better to mention about it in section of past history. For example, a patient presents with complaint of a painless swelling on his fingertip since few days. He informs about the history of pinprick injury at same site few months back. In this case, swelling is most likely to be an "implantation dermoid cyst", which is commonly caused by prick injuries. But since, there is a significant time gap between the injury and the onset of swelling, so it would be better to present the event of pinprick injury in his past history. This is described in details in the next chapter.

Occasionally, some patients correlate the onset of disease with some insignificant and unrelated event. In some cases, this information confuses the student and he even starts thinking in a wrong direction. This is more frequently seen with elderly, rural, and illiterate patients and is more commonly encountered in early stages of student life. For example:

> An old man informs a student about development of a painless swelling in his left inguinal region since 2 months, which he had noticed after taking some medicine from a local doctor for diarrhea and vomiting. Here, his inguinal swelling is likely to be inguinal hernia or lymphadenopathy. Both of them are unlikely to develop because of some medicine. Student was not sure about any correlation and so, he presented the same history to his teacher. Later on, his teacher clarified him that the history of ingestion of medicine is only a coincidental information in this case.

Gradually, the theoretical knowledge and experience of student increase with time and he becomes capable of discriminating between the relevant and irrelevant information from the patients with various types of diseases. Similar problem occurs at few more point of case history, when patient's information cannot be correlated with pathogenesis of disease, e.g., about aggravating or relieving factors of pain, etc. *But whenever in doubt, a student should prefer to include the information for presentation.* It would be better for an undergraduate student to note some insignificant information from the patient rather than to miss any significant point in his case history.

Course of the Disease

This information describes the course of symptoms (and the disease) from their onset till present time.

A symptom may progress, may remain static, or even may regress during course of the disease. The progression may be in terms of severity, frequency, periodicity, size, etc. For example:
- Initially mild pain, later on severe pain
- Initially dysphagia for solid food, later on dysphagia for liquids also
- Initially dyspnea at exertion, later on dyspnea at rest also
- Initially vomiting once in 2-3 days, later on vomiting 2-3 times in a day
- Initially intermittent pain, later on continuous pain
- Initially small swelling/lump/ulcer, later on large swelling/lump/ulcer.

In some cases, mode of progression of a symptom can give a precious clue for the diagnosis. For example, a patient says that his swelling was static for many years, but has started increasing since last few weeks. This type of progression is indicating toward a malignant transformation of some benign tumor.

It is not a rule that all the symptoms essentially progress during the course of illness. Some remain static and some other may even regress also. This may be because of some medicine which has been taken during the illness or simply due to the natural defense mechanism of the body. For example, a swelling caused by some insect bite or a hematoma resulting from some trauma may even regress in size with passage of time with/without any treatment.

Characteristic Features of Symptoms

Every symptom has got certain features which help the doctor in making the diagnosis of the disease. Different diseases present with similar symptoms, but they may have different features. Following are few examples:
- Patients with renal stone complain of dull aching type of abdominal pain while colicky pain favors the diagnosis of ureteric stone.
- A child with neck swelling and high-grade fever is likely to have acute bacterial lymphadenitis while a low-grade fever will go more in favor of tubercular lymphadenitis.
- Abdominal pain which is aggravated by meals but is relieved with empty stomach is due to gastric ulcer. In contrast, pain which is

aggravated with empty stomach and is relieved by meals is more likely because of duodenal ulcer.
- Nonbilious vomiting is mostly due to nonobstructive causes (such as gastritis, meningitis, migraine, etc.) while bilious vomiting indicates obstruction of bowel beyond the opening of common bile duct in duodenum.
- Hematuria before micturition may be because of urethral polyp or hemangioma while hematuria after micturition is mostly because of stone in urinary bladder.

Hence, it is essential to enquire about different features of major symptoms to make a provisional diagnosis of the disease. It is difficult to describe here the various features of common symptoms of diseases affecting different systems of human body, as it would be an exhaustive list. Following are only few examples showing description of some common symptoms:
- *Abdominal pain*: Location, severity (mild/moderate/severe), periodicity (continuous/intermittent), character (throbbing, pricking, colicky, etc.), radiation, aggravating and relieving factors, etc.
- *Vomiting*: Frequency, relation with meals, color of vomitus, projectile or nonprojectile, etc.
- *Fever*: Grade (high/low), periodicity (continuous/intermittent/remittent), association with chills and rigor, etc.

Treatment History

It is quite possible that before visiting to the hospital, patient may have consulted some other doctor for his disease, especially if it is of chronic duration. So, it is essential to obtain the maximum possible information about the previous treatment received by the patient for the same disease. This information is more important for a physician, than for a student, as he has to plan his treatment also.

In some cases, it may be difficult to obtain accurate information of the treatment which the patient has received during the course of his illness. He might have lost the old documents or forgotten to bring them to the hospital (such as prescriptions, investigation reports, discharge card, etc.). Even if available, they may not always provide sufficient information. Moreover, a student has to use only his questionnaire to obtain this information, as *he is not supposed to check patient's documents*. Literacy and intellectual level of patient plays an important role here. An intelligent patient will be able to provide more information about various medical or surgical treatments which he has already received for his disease.

Whenever some patient informs about any previous treatment, student or doctor should encourage and guide him to obtain the maximum possible information. He should ask about it in a language which is easily understood by the patient. Some lay terminologies may be useful to know about some investigations or treatment from uneducated patients. For example, fine-needle aspiration cytology (FNAC) test can be asked as *Sui ki jaanch* (means: test by a needle) and biopsy can be called as *Tukde ki jaanch* (means: test of some piece).

Interestingly, some patients intentionally avoid disclosing about any previous treatment for their illness. Usually, these are the patients who are not satisfied with the old regimen. They are afraid that if the doctor comes to know about it, he may ask them to continue the same. So, to start a fresh regimen from beginning, they may refrain from disclosing the older one. But, this is essential for a doctor to know the details of previous treatment, as it would help him in planning some treatment for the same disease.

Negative History

It is not only the presence of some symptoms which helps in diagnosing a disease. Sometimes, *absence* of some other symptoms is equally helpful in making a provisional diagnosis. For example, appendicitis and ureteric stone are two common differential diagnoses for pain in right iliac fossa region. In such a patient, if one finds presence of additional complaint of burning in micturition and absence of constitutional symptoms, such as fever, anorexia, etc., the diagnosis will go more in favor of ureteric stone than the appendicitis.

During presentation, a list of such relevant symptoms should be presented by the student at the end of the section of history of presenting complaints as the *negative history* (such as *besides, there is no history of fever, nausea, or vomiting during course of illness of the patient*).

But, there can be an endless list of symptoms from which a patient is *not* suffering. The selection of relevant symptoms which should be asked to exclude some other diagnoses depends upon theoretical knowledge of suspected disease. So, it may be difficult in initial stages for the student to select the appropriate symptoms which should be mentioned in negative history, but this selection improves with enhancement of his theoretical knowledge and practical experience.

To select the relevant symptoms, one should focus more toward the symptoms which can be logically correlated to the presenting complaints of the patient. For example:
- For a patient presenting with *chest pain*, it would be appropriate to ask about the other symptoms of cardiorespiratory system, such as dyspnea, palpitation, cough, fever, etc.
- For patients with *abdominal pain*, major attention should be focused on symptoms of gastrointestinal symptoms, such as vomiting, diarrhea, constipation, etc.
- If some patient complains about *headache*, student should ask about the complaints of vomiting, fever, blurring of vision, etc., keeping all possible differential diagnoses in mind.
- If an elderly patient presents with complaint of *increased frequency of micturition*, one should ask him about the other urinary complaints, such as urgency, dribbling, poor stream, etc. Benign prostatic hyperplasia is a common disease of old age which may present with various combinations of these symptoms.

ELICITATION OF HISTORY OF PRESENTING COMPLAINTS

Practically, it is one of the most difficult sections of medical history, especially for medical students because:
- Proper enquiry of various characters of different symptoms needs appropriate theoretical knowledge of different diseases.
- Unlike other sections of format (e.g., profile, past history, personal history, etc.), there are no specific points in this section on which some interview can be conducted. Rather, it is to be asked and presented as a short story.
- It needs the highest degree of understanding between the student and the patient during conversation. First, the patient should understand that what exactly the student wants to know and then the student should understand that what the patient is informing. For example, it needs some experience to ask and interpret about the severity (mild, moderate, severe) and character of pain (e.g., throbbing, pricking, colicky, etc.) from a patient suffering from some painful disease.
- The information is mostly received from the patient in a random way. During presentation of case history, a student has to arrange various information of this section in the form of a systematic and presentable speech.

Following are some suggestions for the students to improve their communication with the patients during this section:

1. How to Ask?

After writing down about various complaints and their duration (as presenting complaints), there are several ways by which a student can start this section. The best one is by asking the patient to describe about his disease *since the beginning*, especially if he is suffering from some chronic disease:

Aap shuruat se apni beemari ke bare me bataiye (please tell me about your disease right from the beginning).

Some patients feel comfortable in describing their disease as a story in their own words and language. They are able to convey most of the relevant information in a single speech. Listen to his story carefully and encourage him to speak more about the disease. Proper nonverbal communication (such as head nodding, eye contact, vocal cues, etc.) will play an important role in encouraging him to reveal more information. Once he finishes his story, ask him about whatever has not been included in his short speech. Finally, narrate him a quick summary of relevant information for confirmation and then note it down.

For example, when a student asked a patient to describe about his abdominal pain, he told him about its location, severity, periodicity, and aggravating factor by himself. The remaining important information (such as character of pain, radiation, relieving factor, etc.) was asked by the student using appropriate questions.

Interestingly, this story is more appropriately described by the patients who have been recently interrogated by some other doctor [e.g., by consultant or residents in outpatient department (OPD)], as they know that what exactly the student wants to know.

It needs some experience and proper knowledge of the subject to make a relevant and presentable story from speech of the patient. This art can be learnt only by interacting with maximum number of patients of different diseases during student life.

On the other end, some patients are unable to present in the form of a proper story if they are asked to describe their disease since its beginning. Either they share only a small part of desired information or they start describing the irrelevant issues in details. Such patients should be asked the specific questions targeted to the individual information about the disease in the form of *one question-one answer* type of conversation. For example, different features of abdominal pain can be obtained from such patients by asking individual questions about its location, severity, periodicity, character, radiation, aggravating or relieving factor, etc.

2. How to Write?

Simultaneous writing is difficult and distracting in this section and should be avoided because of following reasons:
- Unlike other sections, there are no specific points in this section on which the information can be asked and noted down. It is based on the story told by the patient which may not be in a systematic and straightforward form. Simultaneous writing of his story may lead to random arrangement of various features. So, it would be better to first listen to all the features carefully and then to arrange them in a systematic and presentable manner.
- The act of writing brings an unavoidable interruption (of speech and eye contact) during communication with the patients and so, it should be kept to a minimum possible level during conversation. Frequent and prolonged interruptions will make the patient uncomfortable while telling the story of his disease.

So, it would be better to first focus on conversation with the patient then select out all the relevant information, present him a summary for confirmation, and finally note it down.

If your patient is having multiple complaints or a chronic history, prefer to note down significant points of this section (history of presenting complaints) on a rough paper sheet first. It will help you in remembering all the points while rephrasing the summary to the patient. Presentation of summary also gives a pleasant feeling to the patient that his doctor was listening to him carefully. Even during writing the history, keep repeating some questions to the patient intermittently, so that he will feel himself engaged in conversation.

For example, after listening to the details from a patient with venous ulcer, a student presented him its summary as:

So, you have informed me that you developed complaints of pain and swelling in both legs since last 6 months. You were comfortable in morning, but your complaints reached to maximum by evening time. You got some relief only when you laid down with pillow beneath your legs. You took some medicines from the doctor in your village and applied some herbal ointment, but they did not work. And since last 1 month, you developed an ulcer and pigmentation around your left ankle. Right? Would you like to add anything else?

Interaction with the patient in section of "History of presenting complaints"

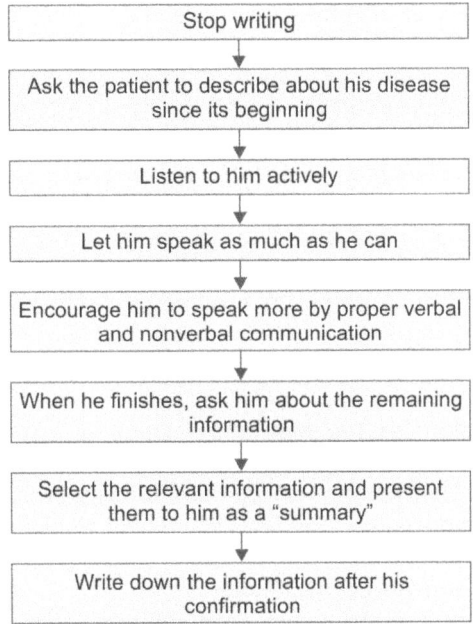

3. Role of Language

The most challenging task for a medical student is to make a presentable speech of "history of presenting complaints" of his patient. In this section, he has to perform following jobs simultaneously:

- *Questioning*: To ask various questions in a language that is easily understood by the patient.
- *Selection*: To select only the relevant information about the disease.
- *Translation*: To translate the information from patient's language to English language.
- *Arrangement*: To arrange the information systematically from beginning till present situation.

In other sections of history, the information is presented on the basis of specific points (e.g. age, religion, hospitalization, appetite, addiction, etc.). But in this section, the student has to present it in form of *short story*, describing the course of disease since beginning. So, a proper knowledge of language plays an important role in writing this section in most presentable form.

It is a well known advice that patient's history should be recorded in his own language. No doubt that the severity of patient's disease can be best described in his own words. But in some cases, it would be better to convert the words in some presentable form. Verbatim translation of spoken words may lead to an unsuitable and bizarre presentation, such as:

- A patient with increased frequency of micturition complains—*mujhe har do-do minute me pishaab karne jana padta hai.*
  Verbatim translation: "My patient has to pass urine in every 2 minutes".
  Interpretation: Increased frequency of micturition.
- A patient with complaint of vomiting describes the volume of vomitus as—*har baar balti bhar ke ulti hoti hai.*
  Verbatim translation: "Every time, he vomits a bucket full of vomitus".
  Interpretation: Profuse vomiting.
- If a patient with complaint of headache informs that—*mujhe aisa lagata hai ki mere sir pe koi haathi baith gaya hai.*
  Verbatim translation: "He feels as if some elephant is sitting on his head".
  Interpretation: Severe headache.

So, a student should not become merely a *translator* who converts every word and sentence of patient in English language. More attention should be paid on interpretation of spoken words rather than simply translating them from one language to another.

No doubt that the students with good knowledge of English language will be able to design and present this section in a better form. But still, others students, who are not very confident and comfortable with English, should not feel it to be a difficult task. Presentation in any language can be very well improved by regular practice.

4. Open-ended Questions versus Closed Questions

The questions which are used for interrogation of any patient can be broadly divided in two different categories:

1. *Open-ended questions:*
   These are unstructured questions which do not suggest any answer and the patient has to reply them in his own words.
   For example:
   - How does your pain aggravate?
   - What was the color of vomitus?
   - Are you suffering from any other problem?

2. *Closed questions:*
   These questions seek very specific reply from the patient and they do not encourage him to provide any additional information. For example:
   - Does your pain aggravate after *walking*?
   - Was the vomitus *brown* in color?
   - Are you suffering from *constipation* also?

   These questions carry a specific answer and so, they give only two options (*yes* or *no*) to the patient.

   As far as possible, closed questions should be avoided while taking history of any patient, especially during early stages. Patient *may not be very sure* while giving any positive or negative answers to these questions.

   The other types of closed questions ask the patient to choose one answer out of a list of the possible options. These questions cannot be replied as *yes* or *no*. But still, they belong to the category of closed questions as they are drawing patient's attention toward some specific answers. For example:
   - How does your pain aggravate? After *walking, running,* or *climbing stairs*?
   - What was the color of vomitus: *green, yellow,* or *brown*?
   - Are you suffering from any other problem, such as *headache, vomiting, or constipation*?

Leading questions: Some questions lead patient's mind toward a fixed direction and they eventually make him feel that the *doctor wants to hear a particular answer from him*. For example:
- Your pain aggravates after walking, does not it?
- You didn't have brown vomiting, did you?
- You are also suffering from constipation, ain't you?

These questions will make the patient think that his doctor wants to hear that his pain aggravates after walking, he never had brown-colored vomiting, and he is also suffering from some constipation. He finds it difficult to contradict these questions and is merely obliged to agree with his doctor's thinking. Such type of questions should never be used during conversation with the patients.

Reliability of any information decreases if it is obtained by asking some closed question or leading question to the patient. In contrast, an open-ended question makes the patient to think about it as it does not guide his attention toward any particular answer. For example:

Gastric ulcer is one of the common differential diagnoses for patients presenting with chronic abdominal pain in epigastric region.

Pain of the gastric ulcer increases with meals and is relieved when stomach is empty. If a physician asks about the aggravating factors of pain as an open-ended question (*aapka dard kaise badta hai?*: How does your pain aggravate?), patient will first think about it and will inform only if his pain certainly aggravates after meals.

In contrast, if he asks about it as a closed question (*kya aapka dard khana khane ke baad badh jata hai?*: Does your pain aggravate after taking meals?), it is quite possible that some patients may incorrectly give a positive reply, even if there is no definite relation of pain with the meals. This information may wrongly lead the physician to think about the possibility of gastric ulcer in such cases.

This relationship of pain with meals will become even less reliable, if the physician asks it as a leading question (*aapka dard khana khane ke baad badh jata hai na?*: Your pain aggravates after taking meals, doesn't it?), as it is almost compelling the patient to give a positive reply.

So, the most reliable information of aggravating factor for pain will be obtained only by using an open-ended question. Patient will give a specific reply to it, only if his pain gets aggravated after taking meals.

Similarly, it would be better to ask the patient to tell about the color of vomitus by himself without suggesting any list of various colors (such as green, yellow, brown, etc.). If he is not very sure, he may be asked to match it with the color of any surrounding object (such as curtains, bed sheet, wall, etc.).

As mentioned earlier, a single disease can present with multiple symptoms of different duration and severity. Information about any other associated problem is best obtained by using some open-ended question. For example:

> A patient with abdominal pain was interrogated by two different types of physicians. Apart from pain, he was also suffering from mild burning in micturition. The first physician asked about the additional complaints in form of an open-ended question (*are you suffering from any other problem?*). Patient thought for a while and informed him about only one additional complaint of burning in micturition. In contrast, the other physician directly used some closed and leading questions for interrogation (*apart from pain, do you feel some nausea or distension of abdomen also?*). Though the patient was not having any such complaints, still he gave him a positive answer. This approach wrongly included few vague and nonspecific symptoms to the list.

Chapter 9: History of Presenting Complaints

But, proper history of the patient may not be obtained by using only the open-ended questions. Sometimes, you may have to use some closed questions also. For example, a patient may forget to inform you about some additional symptoms which are *mild* in intensity and *occasional* in frequency during the course of the disease. For example:

> An elderly female presented to a surgeon with the only complaint of constipation since 6 months. When he asked her about the additional symptoms using open-ended question *(Do you have any other complaints?)*, she said no. But later on, when the surgeon asked her in form of a closed question *(Did you ever have any other problem like blood in your stools?)*, she revealed an additional complaint of occasional rectal bleeding.

A good interrogator uses a proper combination of open-ended and closed questions. *Only open-ended questions should be asked in the beginning while closed questions are usually used as follow-up to open-ended questions.* Also, the interpretation of information obtained by closed questions should be made cautiously.

Following example will help you in understanding the use of different types of questions during communication with your patients:

A patient presented with a swelling in front of his neck. Now, if student wants to know that whether it is painful or painless, there are three different ways in which the question can be framed.

1. *Kya aapko is gathan se koi aur takleef hoti hai?* (Do you have any other complaint with this swelling?)

   This is an open-ended question, as it has not used the word *pain* in it. Now, if the swelling is painful, patient will give a positive reply to this question. But, if his pain is very mild, he may forget to inform you about it, unless you specifically ask him about in form of a closed question, as mentioned below:

2. *Kya aapko is gathan me dard hota hai?* (Do you feel any pain in this swelling?)

   This is a closed question, as it will draw his attention toward the specific complaint of pain. It will reduce the chances of missing any mild or occasional pain. But, it should always be asked only *after* asking an open-ended question, as asked above.

3. *Aapko is gathan me dard bhi hota hai na?* (You feel some pain in this swelling, don't you?)

   This is a leading question, as it may force the patient to give a positive reply only. It should always be avoided during conversation, as it is more likely to give rise to a false positive or exaggerated reply from the patient.

In short, while taking history of any patient, you should prefer to ask the open-ended questions, should use close questions cautiously, but should never ask any leading question.

5. How to Present?

During presentation, the section of history of presenting complaints should begin as (for example): *My patient was apparently alright till 2 months back, when she incidentally noticed a lump in her left breast.*

Here, it is important to use word *apparently*, as it would be wrong to say "My patient was alright", even if he says that he was absolutely fine before that period. Because, it is quite possible that he may be having *some other* major or minor disease, even before occurrence of his presenting illness.

For example, a 60-year-old male presents in surgical OPD with complaint of a nonhealing ulcer on his right foot since 3 months. He is hypertensive since 10 years, diabetic since 2 years, and is suffering from constipation since 1 year. Now, since he is suffering from so many other diseases, it would be incorrect to present him as "alright 3 months back". It would be better to call him "apparently alright 3 months back", which means that before that duration, he was not having the problem which has made him to visit the surgeon at present, i.e., his presenting complaint of nonhealing ulcer.

CHAPTER 10

Past History

> *We never listen when we are eager to speak.*
> —*Francois de la Rochefoucauld*

This section enquires about any significant medical or surgical illness in the past life of the patient. It may or may not have a direct relation with his present illness, but many a times, provides significant information for making the diagnosis or planning management of his current disease.

It includes:
- History of any significant disease
- History of any surgery
- History of hospitalization
- History of any other significant event
- History of similar complaints in the past

GENERAL CONSIDERATIONS

In general, following points should be remembered while enquiring about the past history of any patient:
- Before starting the questionnaire of this section, it would be better if student informs the patient that now he is moving from his present to the past (*"So, it was all about your present illness. Now, I would like to know something about your past life."*).
- The word *past* should not be confused with its dictionary meaning, i.e., *something which has gone by in time and no longer exists.* This section includes both cured as well as current chronic diseases. For example, a patient had suffered from tuberculosis 8 years back, which was cured by proper antitubercular treatment. Now, he is hypertensive at present and taking antihypertensive drugs for last 5 years. Both of these diseases (tuberculosis and hypertension) should be included in his past history.

- The extent to which a patient can recall some event from his past life largely depends on his memory and on the time of its occurrence. For example, an elderly patient may not remember the details of some event (such as hospitalization or surgery) which had happened in his remote past. So, do not force him excessively to recall and provide detailed information about it. If very much required, the details can be obtained from any of his close relatives.
- This chapter includes the *minimum enquiry* which should be made by an undergraduate medical student during history taking whenever a patient gives a positive history of some chronic disease in his past. For detailed questionnaire of common diseases, students are advised to refer any of the standard clinical books of respective subjects.

HISTORY OF ANY SIGNIFICANT DISEASE

Epidemiologically, prevalence of various diseases varies in different parts of the world. Hence, the list of common diseases which should be enquired in this section will differ from place to place. In our country, past history should include an enquiry about common diseases, such as tuberculosis, diabetes, hypertension, asthma, epilepsy, jaundice, etc.

Tuberculosis

Tuberculosis is one of the major chronic diseases in our country which accounts for about one-fifth of the global incidence. It is not confined only to the respiratory system, as tubercular bacilli can affect almost every organ of human body (such as respiratory system, gastrointestinal system, nervous system, reproductive system, etc.). For example:
- A patient presenting with chronic abdominal pain, diarrhea, and weight loss may be a case of *abdominal tuberculosis* (Koch's abdomen).
- A female presenting with infertility may be a case of *tubercular salpingitis*.
- A painless swelling in the neck of a patient may be due to *tubercular lymphadenitis*.
- A child presenting with history of convulsions may be suffering from *tubercular meningitis*.
- Lower limb deformity in an elderly patient may be due to *tuberculosis of hip joint*.

So, regardless of the presenting complaints, it is essential to ask about the past history of tuberculosis to every patient in our country, especially if he is from low socioeconomic class.

Tuberculosis is commonly known to the people as its abbreviation "*TB*". Pure Hindi translations such as *Tapedik rog* or *Kshaya rog* are relatively unknown to most of the people. Patients of all age groups and socioeconomic class very well understand about this disease if been asked as "*TB ki beemari*".

If some patient is unable to understand it by the name of "*TB*", some indirect methods can be used to ask about it, such as:
- Have you ever suffered from *chronic cough* in the past?
- Have you received some *prolonged treatment* (of about 6 or 9 months) in the past?

Any information obtained by these indirect methods should be interpreted cautiously. Any positive reply to such questions should only lead to a *suspicion* of disease. Because, some of the common symptoms of tuberculosis such as chronic cough, low grade pyrexia, weight loss, etc., can be seen in some other diseases also (e.g., chronic bronchitis, bronchogenic carcinoma, etc.).

Tuberculosis is diagnosed only on the basis of proper investigations (such as Mantoux test, sputum examination, X-ray chest, etc.). Occasionally, patients of chronic cough or fever, who do not respond to routine antibiotics, are erroneously diagnosed by quacks as tuberculosis without proper investigations. So, whenever a patient gives history of tuberculosis in past, it is essential for the doctor to know about *who had diagnosed it*. Diagnosis would be more authentic if it was made by some experienced and reliable doctor or center.

Whenever any patient gives a positive history of tuberculosis in past, an enquiry should be made about following information, at least:
- When did he suffer from tuberculosis?
- Did he receive the complete course of antitubercular treatment?

It should be remembered that occasionally, some patients intentionally hide the history of tuberculosis, as they consider it a social stigma. In such cases, indirect methods (as mentioned above) can give some clue about its occurrence in past life of the patient.

Diabetes

Like tuberculosis, diabetes is another common chronic disease which affects multiple systems of the body. It can lead to a wide variety of diseases, such as diabetic retinopathy, diabetic nephropathy, diabetic neuropathy, poor wound healing, diabetic foot, etc. Unlike tuberculosis, which is common in low socioeconomic class, diabetes is more prevalent in middle and high class patients. Still, all patients should be enquired about the history of diabetes, regardless of their presenting complaints and socioeconomic class.

While educated patients call it as *diabetes* or *sugar*, others know it more commonly as *"shakkar ki beemari"* (means: disease of sugar).

If a patient gives a negative reply to your question, he should not be considered as nondiabetic straightway. He may be an asymptomatic patient of hyperglycemia. In such cases, enquire about the last time when he had got his blood sugar level checked. He can be considered as nondiabetic only if his recent blood sugar level was found to be normal. But, if he has never been tested for it or his report was normal many years ago, a fresh blood sugar level test will be required before commenting upon his diabetic status.

Some indirect methods, which are based upon the common symptoms of diabetes, may be helpful in some cases, e.g., history of polyphagia (excessive appetite), polydipsia (excessive thirst), polyuria (excessive urination), poor wound healing, etc. But, like in case of tuberculosis, interpretation should be made cautiously as these features may be caused by some other diseases also (e.g., increased frequency of micturition in benign prostatic hyperplasia, increased appetite by hyperthyroidism, etc.). Moreover, these classical symptoms (polyphagia, polydipsia, and polyuria) are mainly seen in type I diabetes while most of the patients seen in clinical practice are of type II diabetes. So, absence of these features from the history of any patient cannot confidently rule out the possibility of diabetes.

Following information should be obtained from any patient who gives a positive history of diabetes:
- Since how long is he diabetic? It is essential to know about the duration of disease as most of the complications of diabetes develop only after a chronic course of disease.
- What kind of treatment is he taking for it? i.e., is he taking some injection (insulin) or some tablets (oral hypoglycemic drugs)?

Many a times, diabetes has got no role in etiopathogenesis of patient's disease, and so, is not of much importance while making its provisional diagnosis. But, it may play an important role while planning the management of disease. For example:

A 60-year-old male presented to a surgeon with a sebaceous cyst over his shoulder region. Without asking about any history of diabetes, surgeon excised the cyst in minor operation theatre. At the time of follow-up after few days, he was surprised to find him back with an infected wound. It was then only when he came to know that the patient was diabetic. When he asked him that why did not he inform him earlier, the old man blankly said—"Why didn't *you* ask me earlier?"'

So, it is essential to ask about the history of diabetes to each and every patient, especially if his disease needs some major or minor surgical procedure.

Hypertension

Like diabetes, hypertension is another common chronic medical disease which can affect different systems of the body (e.g., stroke, ischemic heart disease, hypertensive retinopathy, etc.). Hence, regardless of his presenting complaints, every patient must be enquired for the history of hypertension, especially if he is middle aged or elderly.

While educated patients can easily understand it as *high BP, high blood pressure* or *hypertension*, others usually know it as "*blood pressure ki beemari*".

Like as in case of diabetes, whenever any patient gives no history of hypertension in his past, it should be enquired that when he had got his blood pressure checked. If it is found that he has never got his blood pressure checked, or if it was normal many years ago, the possibility of him being hypertensive should not be ruled out straightway (as he can be an asymptomatic hypertensive patient).

Whenever a patient gives a positive history of hypertension, he should be asked following questions, at least:
- Since how long is he suffering from hypertension?
- Is he taking regular treatment for it?

Like diabetes, history of hypertension may be more important for management of the disease in some cases, rather than for making a provisional diagnosis. For example:

A 55-year-old male presented with a painless swelling in his inguinoscrotal region. After examining him, the resident doctor diagnosed it as a reducible inguinal hernia. He explained the line of treatment to the patient and admitted him in surgical ward. During preanesthetic checkup, anesthetist found that the blood pressure of patient was highly raised. On asking the details, patient revealed him that he was hypertensive since last few years but was not taking regular treatment for it. He found him unfit for anesthesia and referred him to a physician who started proper antihypertensive medicines. Surgery for inguinal hernia was postponed till his blood pressure was under control. Patient and his relatives were annoyed as his admission could have been avoided if that resident had asked about the hypertension in OPD only.

So, regardless of the presenting complaints, history of hypertension should be essentially asked to every patient who needs some procedure under some kind of anesthesia, especially if he is middle aged or elderly.

■ HISTORY OF HOSPITALIZATION

Hospitalization is a major and unforgettable event of any person's life. In some cases, this information may provide some valuable clue for making a provisional diagnosis of patient's present illness. For example:

A 45-year-old male was admitted with an abdominal lump in right hypochondrial region. On examination, it was found to be hard, nontender, and arising from his liver. On asking about hospitalization in past, he informed that he was admitted in some hospital few years back, for *some problem* related to his liver. This led to a suspicion of *hepatitis* in his past, which supported a provisional diagnosis of *hepatocellular carcinoma* for his abdominal lump.

The information related to previous hospitalization largely depends on the availability of relevant documents (such as investigation reports, discharge card, etc.). Many a times, patient may have lost these documents, especially if it had occurred in his remote past. Sometimes, patients forget to bring the old documents to the hospital, especially if they are of some unrelated disease. This happens more commonly with the patients who are admitted with some emergency condition.

Specific enquiry should be made about some major event (such as blood transfusion) during his hospitalization in past, with a special emphasis on asking about history of any adverse reaction related to it. This information will be helpful during planning the management of his present illness.

Occasionally, patient may inform about hospitalization for some minor illness in past which has got no role in diagnosis of his present illness. For example, a patient with hydrocele informs about hospitalization for diarrhea and vomiting, few years back. Though it does not seem to be significant information for pathogenesis of hydrocele, still one should listen to him carefully while he is informing about this event from his past. Minor and obviously insignificant information can be ignored, but whenever in doubt, it would be better to err on the side of inclusion.

HISTORY OF ANY SURGERY

Like hospitalization, this is another significant event in past life of any patient which may be helpful in planning diagnosis and management of his present disease. For example:
- A patient with features of intestinal obstruction (abdominal distention, bilious vomiting, etc.) gave a history of appendectomy few years back. This guided the surgeon toward a suspicion of postoperative adhesive obstruction.
- An anemic patient informed the doctor about history of gastrectomy in his past which led toward a possibility of pernicious anemia.

Many patients are not able to provide deep details of surgery, especially if it was done in his remote past. Documents may not be available or may not provide the sufficient information. So here also, questionnaire of doctor play an important role in obtaining the details of the surgery.

Whenever a patient informs about any surgery in past, try to get the following information, at least:
- For which disease was he operated?
- When was the surgery performed?
- Was there any significant event in his postoperative period (e.g., wound infection, incisional hernia, etc.)

Some surgeries are commonly noticed in past history of many patients, especially the middle aged and elderly patients (such as cesarean section, tubectomy, vasectomy, cataract surgery, etc.). Other common surgeries in this list are appendectomy, hernioplasty, cholecystectomy, hysterectomy, hemorrhoidectomy, etc.

If a patient informs about some significant event in relation to his previous surgery (e.g., history of difficult intubation, allergy to some drug, etc.), maximum possible attempts should be made to know its details. This could provide some valuable information, especially when some surgical management of his present disease is planned.

HISTORY OF ANY OTHER SIGNIFICANT EVENT

Apart from disease, surgery or hospitalization, history of any other significant event in past life of patient may provide a strong clue for diagnosis in some cases. Following are few examples:

A 10-year-old child presented with a swelling in epigastric region of abdomen. His parents revealed history of blunt abdominal injury while playing in school, few weeks back. This information led to strong suspicion of pseudopancreatic cyst.

A 45-year-old male presented with a painless slowly growing swelling at tip of his right index finger since few days. He was able to recall the history of pin prick injury at same site, few months back. It favored toward a diagnosis of implantation dermoid cyst.

A 5-month-old girl was brought to a surgeon with a nontender swelling on her left thigh. On enquiring about any significant event in past, her parents informed him about history of DPT vaccination at same site, few weeks ago. This information helped the surgeon in making a provisional diagnosis of sterile abscess (post DPT vaccination).

A known case of rheumatic heart disease presented with complaints of fever and malaise. He also gave a history of tooth extraction few days ago. This information helped the physician in suspecting the development of infective endocarditis in his case.

In some cases, a history of visit to some endemic area of disease in past provides a valuable clue for it diagnosis. For example:

In Delhi, a 30-year-old male presented with complaint of painless swelling of his left leg for 1 month. He revealed a history of visit to Bihar, around an year back. This information led to a suspicion of *filariasis* in his case.

Any such major event should be included in the section of past history only if there is significant time gap between the event and the onset of disease. But if the event has occurred just before the onset of disease, it would be better to include it in the section of history of presenting complaints (as described in previous chapter). For example, if a patient develops a swelling on fingertip after few months of needle prick injury, it should be included in his past history. But, if some patient develops swelling and pain of his lower limb after few days of a thorn prick injury, it should be mentioned in the section of history of presenting complaints (in *onset of disease*).

HISTORY OF SIMILAR COMPLAINTS IN PAST

Some diseases are well-known for their recurrent nature. A history of same complaints in past life of the patient may be a valuable information for making a provisional diagnosis of such diseases. Following are few examples:

A patient presented with a swelling on the floor of his mouth. He informed the surgeon about the occurrence of a smaller sized swelling at the same location, few years back. This information helped him in suspecting a diagnosis of *ranula*.

A girl presented with severe pain in right iliac fossa since few hours. She also informed the physician about several episodes of similar pain few months back. This information led him toward a suspicion of *ureteric stone*.

A patient presented with features of intestinal obstruction (abdominal distension, bilious vomiting, etc.). On asking about his past, he informed the surgeon about history of laparotomy for peptic ulcer perforation few years back. Besides, he also informed about the occurrence of similar complaints for several times after his surgery. These two information strongly guided the surgeon toward a diagnosis of *postoperative adhesive obstruction*.

Similarly, some other emergency conditions which may present with a positive history of similar complaints in past are bronchial asthma, epilepsy, migraine, transient ischemic attacks, bleeding in hemophilia, etc.

Previous episodes of same disease may not be of same severity, so, this question should be specifically asked to the patient ("Did you ever suffer from similar complaints in past?"), as sometimes, patient may forget or ignore to inform about the previous episode of same disease, especially if it was of very mild nature.

Previous episodes of similar complaints should be mentioned in past history of the patient only if they have occurred in his *remote past*. If old episodes have occurred recently, it would be more logical to include them in presenting complaints only. For example, compare the history of two patients with complaint of acute pain in right iliac fossa region since few hours. When they were asked about any history of similar pain in past, first patient gave a history of similar episode 6 months back, while the second one informed about two more episodes of similar pain in last 7 days. Now, the previous episode should be mentioned in past history of first case. But it would be more logical to present all episodes of second case in his chief complaints (as complaint of "recurrent abdominal pain since a week".)

CHAPTER 11

Personal History

Think like a wise man but communicate in the language of the people.
—***William Butler Yeats***

The lifestyle of a patient may be the cause of his disease and at the same time, the diseases of a patient may affect his lifestyle.

This section of medical history includes various information which are related to the patient's lifestyle, environment, personal habits, etc. It includes the information about patient's:

- Sleep
- Appetite
- Diet
- Weight change
- Addiction
- Bladder and bowel habits
- Marital status and children

The information obtained in this section may be helpful in following different ways:

- Some information may be valuable for making a provisional diagnosis of patient's disease, e.g., increased sleep and decreased appetite in hypothyroidism, increased appetite in duodenal ulcer, etc.
- Some others show the severity of the disease and its impact on lifestyle of the patient, e.g., decreased sleep in painful conditions, infertility in a man with varicocele, etc.
- Some information helps the doctor in planning the proper management of the disease. For example, it is essential to manage problems, such as constipation and straining in micturition in an elderly patient with inguinal hernia, otherwise it may lead to a recurrence after surgery.

GENERAL CONSIDERATIONS

Following general points should be remembered while enquiring about the personal history of any patient:
- Before starting the questionnaire of this section, it would be better if you inform the patient that you are going to ask about his lifestyle (*So, it was all about your disease. Now, I would like to ask you something about your routine life*). This is essential as the patient with any disease is usually not prepared to get these types of questions from his doctor.
- The relative importance of every point of this section depends on the disease of the patient. What is important for one patient may not have equal importance for the other one. For example, dietary history is important for a patient presenting with a complaint of epigastric pain (e.g., excessive spicy diet may lead to peptic ulcer disease), but the same information is almost useless for another patient with inguinal hernia. An experienced physician knows about the relative importance of different questions for various diseases, but a medical student has to ask all the questions to all types of patients during his training period.
- Some questions of this section may be surprising and absolutely unanticipated for some patients. So, keep yourself prepared for some unusual response from such patients. Occasionally, you may have to explain some curious patient about the reason behind asking such unexpected questions.
- Any change in lifestyle of the patient (e.g., sleep, weight, appetite, etc.) should be considered significant *only if it can be correlated with his present illness*. A change which is physiological (e.g., decreased appetite due to old age) may not be very useful for making provisional diagnosis of the disease. In fact, such information may even confuse and mislead the inexperienced students.

SLEEP

Sleep of a patient can get altered by a large number of conditions; most of them are medical or psychiatric diseases. For example:
- Insomnia (sleeplessness) is seen in anxiety, mania, schizophrenia, hyperthyroidism, etc.
- Hypersomnia (excessive sleepiness) can occur due to hypothalamic disorders, uremia, hypothyroidism, depression, etc.

Besides, some other diseases may indirectly affect the normal sleep pattern of the patient. For example:
- Severely painful diseases may not allow the patient to sleep comfortably, e.g., chronic pancreatitis, peripheral vascular diseases, etc.
- Sleep of a patient with benign prostatic hyperplasia may get disturbed because of increased frequency of micturition during nighttime.
- Some diseases may make the patient uncomfortable in supine position, e.g., gastroesophageal reflux disease, congestive cardiac failure, Buerger's disease, etc. This indirectly affects his sleep as well.

Moreover, it should be remembered that sometimes sleep of a patient may get affected because of the side effects of the medicines for his disease. For example, drugs, such as steroids, theophylline, and beta-blockers can decrease the sleep of the patient while hypersomnia is seen in patients taking antihistaminics, antipsychotics, etc. Also, if a patient is chronic alcoholic, his insomnia may be simply a manifestation of alcohol withdrawal.

If a patient informs about some change in his sleep, it is important to know about the duration since it has changed. Specify the patient that you want to know if there is any change in his sleep after the onset of his disease.

It is quite common to find some sleep disturbance in elderly patients regardless of their chief illness. Reversal of the sleep pattern (nighttime insomnia and daytime somnolence) is commonly seen in the old age.

Occasionally, sleep of some patients gets decreased only after hospitalization. Such a change is of no significance as it can be attributed to many factors other than his disease (e.g., change of sleeping place, lack of physical activity in daytime, etc.).

So, it is very easy to ask any patient about his sleep, but the interpretation should be made cautiously. Any change of sleep pattern cannot always be attributed to his present illness.

APPETITE

Appetite means the *desire to eat food*, which is felt as hunger. A change in appetite of the patient may provide valuable information for making a diagnosis of his disease. For example:
- Appetite is decreased in hypothyroidism, depression, acute appendicitis, gastric ulcer, carcinoma of stomach, tuberculosis, advanced malignancy, etc.

- Increased appetite is seen in diabetes, hyperthyroidism, anxiety, duodenal ulcer, etc.

Like sleep, it is easy to enquire about the appetite of the patient, but proper interpretation of any change needs some precautions. Following points should be remembered while asking about the appetite of any patient:
- Any change in appetite of the patient should be considered significant only if it can be correlated to his disease. The possibility of other causes, which can affect a person's appetite, should be excluded before considering any change as significant.
- Loss of appetite is commonly seen in old age, which should be considered as a part of aging process. Lack of physical activity, inability to chew properly, and decreased taste and smell sensation are some of the common factors responsible for this change. For example, a 60-year-old male patient with inguinal hernia complains of reduced appetite since last few years. Here, this information is positive but insignificant as it has got no role in diagnosis or management of hernia.
- Many diseases can indirectly reduce the appetite of the patient through multiple factors, such as lack of physical activity, adverse effect of some medicine (e.g., acetazolamide, metronidazole, etc.), change of quality of food (from home to hospital), etc. So, even if a patient complains of loss of appetite since the onset of disease, it cannot always be attributed directly to his disease.
- If a patient is unable to inform properly about his appetite, some indirect methods can be used. Most commonly asked question is about the "number of *chapattis* per meal". For example, a patient says that earlier three chapattis were enough for him in the lunch or dinner, but now he feels satiety only after eating five or six chapattis. This change very much indicates toward an increase in his appetite.

This method is quite commonly used for assessment of appetite of patients. It is easy to ask and calculate, but needs some caution during interpretation. There can be some other reasons behind variation in number of chapattis. For example, it may be possible that because of his disease, patient may have developed disliking for chapattis and so, he has increased the amount of other easily digestible food material (e.g., rice) in his meals. So, enquiry should be made by about his *whole meal* and not only about the number of chapattis.

- A change in appetite with *change of weather* is common and physiological (increased in winter and decreased in summer) as it is related to the maintenance of basal metabolic rate of the body.
- In some diseases, patient may have a normal appetite, but may feel *afraid to eat* because of some of his symptoms get precipitated by food (such as pain, vomiting, etc.). For example, pain of gastric ulcer gets aggravated by meals. So, despite of having a desire to eat, a patient with gastric ulcer may avoid food only due to the fear of pain. In such cases, it would be better to call it as sitophobia (food fear) and not the anorexia. In contrast, the appetite of a patient with carcinoma of stomach gets reduced because of true anorexia. Detailed enquiry in suspected cases would reveal the actual cause of decreased appetite.

DIET

Diet of a person is *the kind of food he eats*. It should not be confused with appetite which means his hunger.

Dietary habits of the patient may provide some valuable clue in making the diagnosis or planning the management of some diseases.

Following are some of the common questions to be asked in the dietary history of the patient:
- *Are you a vegetarian or a nonvegetarian?*
  - Constipation and appendicitis are more common in patients who consume a large amount of refined or nonfiber diet (e.g., bread, meat, etc.).
  - Pernicious anemia is more common in vegetarian people (due to deficiency of vitamin B_{12}).
  - Cysticercosis is more commonly seen in people who eat *pork*.
- *What type of food do you like more: spicy or nonspicy?*
  Some diseases are more common in patients who preferably eat spicy food, e.g., peptic ulcer, carcinoma of stomach, etc.
- What *type of salt do you take: iodized or noniodized?*
  Hypothyroidism is more prevalent in people taking noniodized salt.
- *Do you have any disliking for any specific type of food?*
  It may be due to the intolerance of some specific food, e.g., disliking for wheat products in patients of gluten enteropathy.

The extent of the dietary information to be asked to any patient depends mainly upon his disease. Generally, first two questions are commonly asked by the students from all types of patients, i.e., "vegetarian or nonvegetarian" and "spicy or nonspicy" diet. While superficial questioning is sufficient in most of the patients, detailed enquiry may be required in some cases. For example:

- Constipation is more common in nonvegetarian people, but it is also important to know that *what proportion of his total diet is formed by nonvegetarian food*. Because, if he eats nonvegetarian food very occasionally (e.g., once in a month), his constipation cannot be strongly attributed to his nonvegetarian diet only. So, simply refraining him from nonvegetarian food will not lead to any significant improvement in his constipation.
- In a suspected case of cysticercosis, it becomes essential to enquire that *what type of nonvegetarian food is eaten by the patient?* Because, most of the Indian nonvegetarian people eat mutton, chicken, or fish while the parasite of cysticercosis (*Taenia solium*) is transmitted to humans mainly through improperly cooked *pork.*

Most of the educated patients understand the words *vegetarian* and *nonvegetarian* easily. Others may be asked by giving some examples of commonly consumed nonvegetarian food, such as meat, fish, etc. For example, *do you eat only vegetables or do you eat meat or fish also?*

It is quite common to find a people who eat only the eggs but no animal flesh. It is matter of social debate that whether an egg-eating person is a vegetarian or nonvegetarian. Since most of the above mentioned diseases are related to animal flesh (and not to the egg), from the point of view of medical history, such a person can be considered as a vegetarian only. In true sense, he should be called as an *ovovegetarian* (*eggitarian* is an informal word and so, should not be used for medical records and communications).

This enquiry should be made very cautiously if the patient belongs to the communities which are known for their strict vegetarian food practice (e.g., Brahmins, Jains, etc.). A careless, casual, and straightforward questioning should be avoided in such cases. A strictly vegetarian patient may feel disgusted on being asked bluntly about the nonvegetarian diet.

WEIGHT CHANGE

This section is commonly known as *weight loss*, but it would be better to call it as *weight change* as both increase and decrease of body

weight of a patient may indicate toward some significant disease. For example:
- Some diseases lead to unusual weight loss, such as tuberculosis, malignancy, acquired immunodeficiency syndrome (AIDS), inflammatory bowel diseases, hyperthyroidism, etc.
- Some diseases lead to unusual gain of weight, such as hypothyroidism, renal failure, Cushing's syndrome, polycystic ovarian disease, etc.

Following points should be remembered while assessing any change in weight of the patient:
- Like in cases of sleep and appetite, any physiological cause of weight change should be kept in mind while making the assessment. Interpretation of any change should be made cautiously; otherwise, this finding may mislead the diagnosis in a wrong direction. For example:

> A 60-year-old male presented with a painless swelling in his left scrotum since 2 years, which was irreducible, fluctuant, and transilluminant. He also gave the student a history of some weight loss in last few years. Though the case was having all the classical symptoms and signs of *hydrocele*, still the student was confused with the possibility of *testicular tumor*, only because of the positive history of weight loss.

- Any change in weight is more likely to be significant if a major change has occurred in a short duration, especially after onset of the other symptoms of the disease. This type of finding is more in favor of some pathological cause rather than the physiological change.
- Some patients may wrongly call the other symptoms, such as fatigue or weakness as weight loss. A disease may make a patient feel quite weak without causing actual weight loss.
- Occasionally, history of unusual weight gain since the onset of the disease may be a side effect of some *medicine* being taken for that disease, e.g., steroids, antidepressants, etc.
- Assessment of any change in weight is quite easy if the patient knows his previous and present body weight, but problem arises when patient is not aware of his body weight. In such cases, some indirect methods can be used to get some information. For example:
    - An idea about change in waist circumference can be obtained by asking about any change in the fitting of the patient's *trousers*.

- A change in midarm circumference should be suspected if a female patient is informing about some change in the fitting of her *blouse*.
- Apart from clothes, fitting of ornaments, such as *bangles* and *rings* can be used as an indicator of change in patient's weight.
- Sometimes, relatives of the patient may provide some valuable information about any change in his weight or appearance. Interpretation of some distant relative or unrelated visitor, who has seen the patient after a long time, is more reliable.

ADDICTION

Compulsive physiological and psychological need for a habit-forming substance (such as tobacco, alcohol, etc.) is known as addiction. In a medical history, a detailed enquiry about the patient's addiction may sometimes provide some valuable information for diagnosis and management of his disease.

Following points should be remembered while asking about the addiction of any patient:
- Whenever some patient gives a positive history of any addiction, following additional information should be obtained from him, at least:
  - Since how long is he addicted to it?
  - What is the frequency and amount of addictive substance consumed by him?

    The extent of enquiry depends upon disease of patient and the role interrogator (i.e., physician or student). While superficial enquiry of addiction is sufficient for a medical student, a physician may have to obtain the detailed information for planning the management of disease.

    It is essential to know about the duration of addiction because most of the diseases develop only after chronic consumption of some addictive substance. For example:

> Two patients presented with complaint of hematemesis to a physician. Both gave a positive history of alcohol consumption. On further enquiry, it was found that the first patient was taking two to three pegs of whisky every day since the last 10 years. In contrast, the second one was drinking only one or two pegs occasionally not more than two or three times in a year. On the

Contd...

Contd...

> basis of these details, he strongly suspected *esophageal varices* (due to portal hypertension caused by alcoholic cirrhosis) in the first patient, but started seeking for some other cause of hematemesis for the second one.

- Some patients may feel uncomfortable and embarrassed in accepting about any addiction in front of their relatives. For example, an adolescent boy may not reveal the true history of addiction in front of his parents. So, it would be better not to ask about it openly in a loud voice. If very much suspected, enquiry should be made again in alone away from his family members and relatives.

  Conversely, in some other suspicious cases, an enquiry should be made by the physician from the relatives also in the absence of the patient (*third party history*). For example:

  > A 45-year-old male presented with complaint of severe pain in epigastric region of abdomen. He refused for any type of addiction, but the physician preferred to reconfirm about it from his wife. As he was suspected, she revealed about his habit of alcohol consumption since last few years. This helped the physician to make a provisional diagnosis of acute pancreatitis in his case.

- A literate patient from middle- or high-class family can be directly asked using words, such as *addiction, smoking, drinking,* etc. In contrast, illiterate and low-class patients can be asked by giving the examples of common addictive substances, such as "any habit of *bidi, tambakoo, sharaab,* etc.". Pure Hindi translation of the word addiction (*vyasan*) is not understood by many patients. Words, such as *nasha* or *buri aadat* (bad habit) should be better avoided during conversation with the patients.
- In our country, it is comparatively uncommon to find the addiction of common addictive substances (such as smoking, alcohol, etc.) in female population. So, they should be asked about it very cautiously. It would be better to avoid using words, such as *bidi, tambakoo* (tobacco), or *sharaab* (alcohol) while taking history of female patient. Instead of them, some milder substances, such as *paan* (betel squad) or *supaari* (betel nut) should be used for reference of addiction.
- It is important to know about the duration since the patient is addicted to some substance, but it may be difficult to find in some

cases. Many elderly patients are unable to recall the exact age of starting consumption of some addictive substance. In such cases, it can be presumed that they might have started it from the age of 15-20 years. For example, if a 55-year-old male patient says that he has been addicted to bidi smoking since his *childhood*, he should be considered to be "addicted since about 40 years".

Following are some of the common addictions seen in the patients of our country:

Smoking

This is one of the most common addictions seen in people of our country. One study concluded that about 15% of Indian population of more than 15 years of age has smoked tobacco sometime in their life. Contrary to the belief of a layperson, the hazards of smoking are not limited only to the respiratory system. It can lead to various respiratory diseases, such as bronchiectasis, carcinoma of lung, chronic obstructive pulmonary disease (COPD), etc., as well as the diseases of other systems like ischemic heart disease, peripheral vascular diseases, etc. Besides, tobacco contains many carcinogens which play an important role in etiopathogenesis of many malignancies like that of oral cavity, esophagus, stomach, kidney, urinary bladder, etc. So, it is essential to enquire about the history of smoking to every patient regardless of his presenting complaints.

In our country, tobacco is commonly smoked in the following forms:

- *Bidi smoking:* Addiction of bidi smoking is commonly seen in villagers and urban poors of our country as it is cheaper than the cigarettes. It is around 10 times more commonly smoked than the cigarettes and it accounts for about half of total tobacco consumption in our country. Though it contains less amount of tobacco, still it is more hazardous than cigarettes as it does not contain a *filter* and so, the smoker is exposed to a higher amount of nicotine and carbon monoxide. It is available in different types of packets, which are commonly called as *bundle* by the patients. One bundle of bidi contains about 20-24 bidis inside. On an average, an Indian bidi smoker smokes around 15-20 bidis per day.
- *Cigarette smoking:* In contrast to bidi, cigarette smoking is commonly seen in middle and high classes of urban population of our country. Almost all cigarettes available in the market contain a filter at their tail end. A standard packet of cigarette contains 10 cigarettes inside.

- *Others:* Other less common forms of tobacco smoking in our country are *hookah* smoking (commonly seen in villagers) and pipe or cigar smoking (mostly seen in high-class patients).

Tobacco Chewing

Apart from smoking, this is another popular form of consuming tobacco in our country. This history is more important in cases of patients presenting with some oral or oropharyngeal pathology as chewable tobacco may lead to some major diseases, such as oral cancer, laryngeal cancer, submucous fibrosis, etc.

Chewable tobacco is commonly available in market in two different forms:

1. Dried and crushed leaves of tobacco (*tambakoo*) are mixed with slaked lime (*chuna*) and the mixture is chewed as quid (popularly known as *khaini*). It can also be taken with areca nut (*supari*) or betel leaf (*paan*). This form is more commonly consumed by rural and elderly people.
2. Small pieces of beetle nut are coated with powdered tobacco and flavoring agents. This is popularly known as *Gutkha* or *Pouch* and is more commonly consumed by urban and young population.

In case of addiction of chewable tobacco, enquiry should be made about the duration of addiction and amount of tobacco consumed per day (e.g., by asking number of pouches). Also, it should be asked that whether he has got a habit of chewing tobacco at nighttime. Keeping the tobacco in cheek pouch overnight (*night quid*) increases the risk of carcinoma by several folds.

Alcohol

Alcoholism is one of the common addictions throughout the world. Chronic consumption of alcohol can lead to diseases involving multiple systems of body, such as gastritis, pancreatitis, hepatitis, cirrhosis, peripheral neuropathy, Korsakoff's psychosis, and many more.

In social terminology, the word alcohol is used for all ethanol containing beverages which are used for recreational purpose. Commonly used alcoholic beverages in our country can be divided in two different groups:

1. *Country-made liquor:* It is popularly known by various names, such as *Desi sharab* or *Desi daroo*. It is cheaper but more hazardous and

is commonly consumed by poor and low socioeconomic class patients. The term *Kachchi sharab* is usually used for the liquor prepared by fermenting *mahuwa* flowers and is usually consumed by tribal population.
2. *Indian-made foreign liquor (IMFL)*: This is an official term used by the government and includes different types of western style hard liquors which are manufactured in our country (e.g., beer, rum, whisky, vodka, etc.). They are costlier than country-made liquor and hence are commonly consumed by middle and high socioeconomic class patients. They all differ in concentration of ethanol and different people prefer to consume different types of IMFLs.

In case of history of alcohol consumption, an enquiry should be made about the duration, amount, and type of alcohol consumed. It is easier to estimate the amount of ethanol consumed in cases of IMFL as each type contains a standard concentration of ethanol. The consumed volume can be informed by the patient in terms of *pegs* or *bottles*. One *large peg* contains 60 mL of beverage while a *small peg* means 30 mL. Similarly, a *quarter* contains 180 mL (3 pegs), *half* bottle means 375 mL (approximately 6 pegs), and *full* bottle contains 750 mL (approximately 12 pegs) of IMFL. For example, if a patient informs that he is consuming 2 pegs of vodka every day since last 10 years, it means that he is drinking 120 mL of vodka per day.

Other Addictive Substances

Some other uncommon addictive substances, which are consumed by people of our country, are:
- Ganja (*Cannabis*/marijuana): It is commonly consumed by burning and inhaling the smoke, popularly known as *chillum*.
- Bhang: It is obtained from leaves and flowers of *Cannabis* plant which is consumed as *Bhang goli* or *Munakka* or with milk as *Thandaai*.
- Opium (*afeem*): Commonly consumed by smoking.
- Other narcotic drugs: Like cocaine, heroin, brown sugar, etc.

BLADDER AND BOWEL HABITS

Any change in normal bladder or bowel habits of a patient can sometimes provide valuable information in diagnosis and management of some diseases. Commonly observed bowel problems are constipation, diarrhea, bleeding per rectum, etc., while common urinary complaints are increased frequency, poor stream, dribbling, etc.

It is not essential that alteration in bladder or bowel habits of any patient is caused only by some disease of gastrointestinal or urinary system. It may be a manifestation of some other systemic disease, e.g., constipation in hypothyroidism, diarrhea in hyperthyroidism, etc.

The bladder and bowel habits of any patient should be asked in a language which is easily understood by him.

Seasonal variation in frequency of micturition (increased in rainy season and decreased in summer season) is quite common and physiological.

Some degree of change in bowel habits is common and can be considered as physiological in elderly people. Many old-aged male patients have some urinary complaints (such as increased frequency, urgency, hesitancy, etc.) due to benign enlargement of prostate. So, apart from the chief complaints, most of the elderly patients usually complain of some problem related to their bladder and bowel habits also.

> An elderly female with a lump in her breast since 3 months informed a student about her constipation since 10 years. Though she was admitted in hospital for her breast lump, but still she went in deep details while describing about the constipation. The student was unable to decide the significance of constipation in a case of breast lump. In fact, he got confused that what was her actual complaint: breast lump or constipation?

Sometimes, the information of bladder and bowel habits is more valuable in planning the management of disease of the patient. For example:

> An elderly patient presented to a surgeon with a reducible inguinal hernia. Additionally, he was having some degree of constipation also, but he forgot to inform about it to the surgeon, who missed to ask the bladder and bowel habits of the patient. His surgery was uneventful, but he continued to strain for defecation in postoperative period, which led to a recurrence of hernia after sometime.

MARITAL STATUS AND CHILDREN

Following are some examples where marital history of patient plays an important role in the diagnosis and management of his disease:
- Matrimonial disharmony may lead to some psychiatric disorders, such as depression.
- Counseling and proper investigations of spouse should be done in cases of sexually transmitted diseases (such as AIDS, syphilis, etc.).
- Proper counseling of couple is required in cases of genetic disorders. If one or both of them are suffering from some genetically transmitted disease (e.g., thalassemia, sickle cell anemia, etc.), they should informed properly about the risk of its transmission to their offspring.
- Females with some cardiovascular diseases (such as tetralogy of Fallot, coarctation of aorta, etc.) may not be able to tolerate the physiological stress of pregnancy and delivery. So, proper counseling and special precautions are required in such cases.
- This history is especially important in the diseases which may lead to infertility of the patient. For example:

> A 30-year-old male patient presented with a painless scrotal swelling since a long duration. He was married since 6 years, but was not having any children. This information favored a suspicion of *varicocele* which can cause azoospermia and infertility.

Superficial enquiry of marital status is sufficient in most of the cases. In general, following questions should be asked in this section:
- Is he/she married?
- If yes, since how many years?
- Is he/she having any child/children?
- If yes, what is his/her/their age?

If the patient is a widow/widower or divorced, it should be specifically mentioned in the section of his/her marital status.

It may be difficult for an elderly patient to recall exact age of all of his children, especially if he/she is having a large family. Students should avoid any undue emphasis in obtaining this information. In such a case, it would be sufficient to know about the age of only the elder most and the youngest child of the patient.

CHAPTER 12

Family History

Two monologues do not make a dialogue.
—*Jeff Daly*

In the simplest way, a family can be defined as a group of people sharing the common ancestry. Family history of a patient means an enquiry about the occurrence of same or any other significant disease to any other member of the patient's family.

Following are some examples which show the importance of family history in planning diagnosis and treatment of the disease:

- Many diseases tend to run among the members of family through heredity transmission (e.g., thalassemia, hemophilia, breast cancer, gastric cancer, etc.). A positive family history in such cases can strongly support their diagnosis. For example:

> A 25-year-old female presented with a small painless nodule in her left breast. The surgeon was thinking it to be benign until she gave a history of carcinoma breast to her mother. Appropriate investigations were done and the nodule was found to be malignant.

- Sometimes, a positive family history of some different, but significant disease can give an important clue for diagnosis of disease of the patient. For example:

> An 18-year-old male presented with history of a nonhealing ulcer on his foot. He was not diabetic, but gave a positive history of diabetes in some members of his family. This information raised a suspicion to the doctor. He got his blood sugar level checked, which was found to be raised.

Genetically related relatives (commonly known as *"blood-related persons"*) can be divided in following three groups:

1. *First-degree relatives:* Includes parents, siblings, and offspring (i.e., mother, father, real brother, real sister, son, and daughter)

2. *Second-degree relatives:* Includes grandparents, uncle, aunt, nephew, niece, and grandchildren (i.e., *dada, dadi, nana, nani, chacha, mama, bua, mausi, bhateeja, bhateejee, bhanja, bhanjee, pota, poti, naati,* and *naatin*).
3. *Third-degree relatives:* Includes first cousin, great grandparents, and great grandchildren (i.e., cousin brother, cousin sister, *par-dada, par-dadi, par-pota, par-poti,* etc.).

The easiest way to ask about the family history to any patient is as— "Is any other member of your family suffering from same or any other major disease?". But sometimes, the word *family* draws patient's attention toward the group of people living under the same roof. But, it is not necessary that all people living in the same home are genetically related to each other. For example, in a typical family of three generations (such as a couple with their parents and children), the husband is genetically related to everyone except to his wife. At the same time, wife is genetically related to no one except her children. Occasionally, this confusion can lead to an error of interpretation as shown in following examples:

> A 35-year-old female with a lump in her breast informed a student that her mother-in-law had suffered from carcinoma breast few years back. During presentation, he presented this information as a "positive family history" in favor of the diagnosis. His point was rejected because this cannot be considered as a positive family history, as patient's mother-in-law is not related to her genetically.

> A 25-year-old female presented with complaints of increased appetite and thirst. When student asked her about the health status of other members of her family, she did not inform any significant problem with her husband, children, and in-laws. But, she missed to inform about her elder brother, who was living in her parent's home and was a known case of diabetes mellitus.

So, it will be better to frame the question in an expanded form: "Is any other member of your family, *such as your parents, brother or sister,* suffering from same or some other significant disease?". This will draw patient's attention only toward his/her genetically related relatives, even if they are living miles away from him/her.

If any of the parents or close relatives of the patient are dead, an enquiry should be done to know about the cause of death. This information may provide a valuable clue in some cases. For example:

> An elderly patient presented with a lump in his epigastric region. Both of his parents were dead. On asking about the cause of death, he informed that his father had developed a lump in his abdomen and had suffered from huge abdominal distension in his last days. This suggested a possibility of some intra-abdominal tumor leading to malignant ascites in terminal stages.

HISTORY OF CONTACT

Some diseases are contagious in nature, i.e., they are transmitted from one person to another by direct or indirect contact (e.g., tuberculosis, scabies, worm infestation, hepatitis A, etc.). So, it would be important to know about the history of same disease to any other member of the family. But in such cases, the enquiry should include about all the members (genetically related as well as unrelated) of family of patient. For example, if a female with complaints of cough and fever informs about history of tuberculosis to her mother-in-law, the information carries some significance in making a diagnosis. But in true sense, this cannot be called as a positive family history. It should be called as a positive *history of contact.*

The enquiry of contact in suspected contagious diseases should extend even beyond the boundaries of family, i.e., up to neighborhood, school, working place of patient, etc. Moreover, any information carries some significance only if there was some actual contact of the patient with infected person. For example:

> A 3-year-old child was admitted with complaints of fever and convulsions. His parents gave a history of tuberculosis to his grandfather who had died of the disease 5 years back. Here, this information does not carry much significance as the child had never been in contact with his grandfather.

Similarly, when there is a suspicion of some sexually transmitted disease (such as AIDS, syphilis, etc.), it is important to know about the health status of the spouse also. In such cases, an enquiry should be made about any history of some recent unprotected sexual intercourse with any person other than the spouse of the patient. Such questions should be asked very cautiously, only when there is a strong suspicion of some sexually transmitted disease. A careless and straightforward questioning by some inexperienced young medical student may sometimes lead to an unpleasant and embarrassing situation.

CHAPTER 13

Menstrual and Obstetric History

Words are, of course, the most powerful drug used by mankind.
—*Rudyard Kipling*

This section of medical history is the most important for patients presenting with some obstetric or gynecological complaints. But still, it is essential to ask about it to every female patient as it can provide valuable information for diagnosis and management of the diseases of other systems also. For example:
- Menstrual abnormalities (e.g., menorrhagia, amenorrhea, etc.) can be a manifestation of some endocrinological disorders, such as diabetes, hypothyroidism, hyperthyroidism, etc.
- History of recurrent abortion can be noticed in patients with endocrinological disorders, such as hypothyroidism, diabetes, etc.
- A breast lump in a middle-aged female is more likely to be malignant if she is nulliparous.
- Excessive blood loss in menstruation may be the actual cause in some females presenting with features of anemia.
- Psychiatric diseases, such as depression, anxiety, and sleep disturbance are some of the common symptoms in postmenopausal period.

So, the enquiry of menstrual and obstetric history cannot be restricted only to the patients presenting with obstetric or gynecological diseases. Some superficial questions should be asked to every female patient, regardless of her presenting complaints.

■ MENSTRUAL HISTORY

This includes an enquiry about the following information:
- *Age at menarche:* Menstrual cycle (MC) of a female starts at the age of around 10–15 years (average: 13 years). Early onset can occur in diseases, such as pituitary tumors, ovarian tumors,

hypothyroidism, etc., while late onset of menarche can be seen in hyperthyroidism, diabetes, anemia, malnutrition, etc.
- *Last menstrual period (LMP):* The importance of asking about the LMP to any female patient of childbearing age has been described ahead in this chapter.
- *Length and periodicity of MC:* The duration of menstruation and the number of days between two cycles vary from person to person. For example, normal range of duration of menstrual period is 2–7 days with an average of 4 days. Similarly, the gap between two menstrual cycles can range from 21 to 35 days with an average of 28 days. Any deviation from the normal pattern in a female may indicate toward some underlying gynecological or nongynecological disease, such as hypothyroidism, hyperthyroidism, etc.

  A fraction notation can be used to summarize the information of duration and periodicity of menstruation. For example, *5/28* means that her menstruation occurs in every 28 days and each period continues for 5 days.
- Any problem associated with menstruation (e.g., pain, excessive bleeding, etc.).
- *Age at menopause:* Usually, menstruation of female stops permanently at around 45–55 years (average: 50 years). Early menopause may occur in some gynecological (e.g., premature ovarian failure) as well as nongynecological diseases (such as tuberculosis, diabetes, hypothyroidism, etc.). Delayed menopause may be seen in cases of endometrial carcinoma, uterine fibroid, etc.

Following points should be remembered while enquiring about menstrual history of any female patient:
- Menstruation is a physiological but personal phenomenon for any female person. Any patient would be more comfortable in talking about her menstruation, if the medical student or doctor asks her about it in a confident but gentle manner. Unlike other information, it cannot be discussed openly with every female patient. Her privacy should be respected by avoiding an open and loud questioning of this section.
- Normal pattern of menstruation (duration of cycle and interval between two periods) differs in different females. Duration of 4 days and interval of 28 days are only the average values. It is essential to know about the normal pattern of the patient because abnormality is indicated by any *deviation from the normal pattern.* For example, a female informs that her menstrual period occurs in every 3 weeks and lasts for 7 days. Now, if she is having almost

same pattern of menstruation since its beginning, this cannot be considered as an abnormal finding.
- Some irregularities of menstruation are common around perimenopausal period and can be considered as physiological.
- Most of the educated females call menstruation as *period* or MC while others know it by various local names, such as *mahavaari, maheena, maasik,* etc.
- Different types of words and questions are used in different parts of our country to enquire about various points, such as menarche, LMP, etc. For example, at many places, there is a custom of washing hair on the last day of menstruation. So, the information of the LMP can be obtained from such patient by asking that *when did she wash her hair for last time.* Similarly, in some families, females avoid entering the kitchen during menstrual period. So, menarche of any adolescent female can be informed by her mother by saying that *she has started staying away from the kitchen.*

Importance of Last Menstrual Period

The information of the LMP is important while estimating duration of pregnancy and expected date of delivery (EDD) of any pregnant female.

EDD = First day of LMP + 9 months and 7 days

The enquiry of LMP of any female should not be restricted only to obstetric cases as sometimes it provides a valuable clue in diagnosis and management of other diseases as well. Following are few examples:
- *To make a diagnosis:* The information of LMP helps in making a provisional diagnosis in some cases. For example:

> A 16-year-old unmarried girl presented to a surgeon with a complaint of severe pain in the right iliac fossa region. Her family physician had referred her with a provisional diagnosis of acute appendicitis. When the surgeon asked her about the LMP, she informed with hesitation that she has missed one menstrual period. When he enquired further in the absence of her parents, she gave a history of recent unprotected sexual intercourse with her boyfriend. This information made him to suspect some other diagnoses. Ultrasonography of abdomen was performed which detected ruptured *ectopic pregnancy.* On this basis, surgeon referred her to a gynecologist for further management.

- *To plan the investigations:* This information also helps in planning suitable investigations in some cases. For example:

> A 24-year-old married female presented with complaints of pain in right iliac fossa and burning in micturition. She also gave a history of a small stone in her right kidney which was diagnosed few months back. The doctor strongly suspected for ureteric calculus and sent her for an X-ray of kidney, ureter, and bladder (KUB) region. Unfortunately, he had missed to ask her about the LMP. This mistake did not reveal the important information of one *missed period.* She was pregnant and the developing fetus was accidentally exposed to the radiation and its teratogenic effects. Though she was also suspicious of her pregnancy (because of missed period), but she had not informed the doctor about it as she was absolutely unaware of the hazards of radiation exposure during pregnancy.

So, never forget to rule out the possibility of pregnancy before sending any female of childbearing age for an investigation which leads to radiation exposure (e.g., X-rays, CT scan, etc.).

Similar precaution should be taken while prescribing any new drug to female patients of childbearing age as many drugs are well known for their teratogenic potential (e.g., streptomycin, valproic acid, etc.). Negligent prescription may lead to various congenital anomalies and even to the miscarriage of the fetus.

If any female of reproductive age group has missed her menstrual period, the possibility of pregnancy should be confirmed or ruled out by appropriate investigations [e.g., urine pregnancy test, serum human chorionic gonadotropin (hCG), etc.]. If positive, it would be better to prefer some safer investigations (e.g., ultrasonography of abdomen) or other alternative drugs which do not have any harmful effect on the developing fetus.

Rule of ten: It is a well-known rule that *every female with secondary amenorrhea should be considered to be pregnant unless proved* otherwise. But, there is no rule which says: "no amenorrhea-no pregnancy".

In other words, pregnancy should be ruled out first whenever any female of reproductive age gives a history of missed period, but at the same time, it is quite possible for a female to be pregnant *without* any history of amenorrhea. For example:

> A 24-year-old married female visits to a doctor on 4th August with some complaints. Her LMP had started on 10th July and average duration between her two menstrual periods is around 30 days. Now, since she is expecting her next period to start on around 9th August, she will not give any history of amenorrhea on 4th August. But the fact is that she has already conceived in the middle of her present cycle (i.e., around 24th July, as ovulation occurs around 14th day of a normal MC). So, though there is no history of amenorrhea, presently she is pregnant with an 8–10-day-old developing embryo inside her uterus.

Hence, it would be dangerous to rule out the pregnancy confidently only on the basis of history of amenorrhea. To avoid this mishap, one should follow the *rule of ten*, which recommends that it is safer to expose any female of childbearing age to radiation or drug during *first 10 days from her last menstruation*. In other words, first half of MC is comparatively safer for any such exposure than the second one. For example, in above mentioned case, her next menstruation will occur from 10th to 13th August. So, it would be safer to expose her to some drug or radiation from 13th to 23rd August only (i.e., in preovulatory phase of her MC).

Following are some important instructions related to selection of proper investigation for females of childbearing age:
- Pregnancy should be confirmed or ruled out by appropriate investigation (e.g., urine test). The doctor can safely proceed with such investigations, if the test is found to be negative.
- If one cannot rule out pregnancy instantly by some tests, *safer* investigations (e.g., ultrasonography of abdomen, instead of X-ray) and drugs should be preferred for such patients. It is always better to be safe than sorry.
- If possible, investigations involving radiation exposure (e.g., X-ray, CT scan, etc.) should be postponed to the safer period, as described by the rule of ten. For example, if the above mentioned female has visited on 4th August with some nonurgent complaint (e.g., chronic backache), it would be safer to call her for an X-ray anytime from the beginning of her next menstruation (around 9th August) to 22nd August.
  - *To plan the treatment:* In some cases, the information of LMP helps the doctor in planning some surgical treatment of the patient. For example:

Chapter 13: Menstrual and Obstetric History

> A 35-year-old female patient was admitted to a surgical ward with third-grade hemorrhoids. She was planned for a routine surgery in the next 2–3 days. While taking her history in the outpatient department (OPD), the resident doctor had forgotten to ask about her LMP. When another resident in the ward enquired about it, he found that her next menstrual period was likely to commence in the next 3–4 days. On this basis, her surgery was postponed for about 10 days. Routine surgeries of pelvic region should be avoided during menstrual period of any female patient.

Hence, it is valuable to know about the LMP of any female patient of childbearing age regardless of her presenting complaints. It should be enquired from both obstetric and nonobstetric cases.

OBSTETRIC HISTORY

This section includes information related to previous pregnancies and deliveries of the female patients. It is commonly recorded using *gravida/para/abortus (GPA) system* as follows:

- *Gravida*: It indicates the number of times a female has become pregnant in her life.
  This is irrespective of outcome of previous pregnancies. In other words, it includes all pregnancies regardless of whether they led to childbirth or medical termination or spontaneous abortion, etc. A *primigravida* is a female who has become pregnant for the first time while *multigravida* is the one who has become pregnant in the past for two or more times.
- *Para*: It indicates the number of pregnancies which were carried beyond the period of viability of fetus. As per Indian standard, period of viability is considered as 28 weeks. This is irrespective of final outcome of pregnancies, i.e., whether they led to live birth or stillbirth. Any pervious pregnancy, which was continued beyond 28th week, should be included in it.
  A *nullipara* is a female who has never carried a pregnancy beyond 28th week while a *multipara* is the one who has carried previous pregnancies beyond 28th week for two or more times regardless of whether baby was born alive or not.
  Students should not confuse *para* for the number of children. For example, a female gives a history of becoming pregnant twice in the past but unfortunately, both the pregnancies had resulted in

stillbirth only. Now, though she is not having any offspring, she would still be considered as a multipara as both of her pregnancies were continued beyond the period of viability.
- *Abortus (or abortion)*: It indicates the number of pregnancies which were lost due to any reason (such as induced abortions, spontaneous abortion, etc.). Stillbirths are not included in this category.

In practice, two additional information are included in this system.
- *Living children*: Total number of living children of female at present time.
- *Dead children*: Total number of children who died after birth at any age due to any cause. Stillbirths are included in this category.

Besides, the enquiry of mode (vaginal/assisted/cesarean) and outcome (full term/preterm/stillbirth) of previous deliveries should be made in obstetric history of the patient. In case of history of previous cesarean section, an attempt should be made to know about its indication also. Fetal distress, abnormal presentation, prolonged labor, etc., are some of the common indications of cesarean section in routine practice.

For writing purpose, obstetric history of any female patient is usually abbreviated as G, P, A, L, and D. For example, a 32-year-old pregnant female gives following information about her obstetric history:
- *At 20 years*: She became pregnant for the first time, but it was terminated medically in first trimester.
- *At 21 years*: Her second pregnancy led to a spontaneous abortion in first trimester.
- *At 23 years*: She gave birth to a healthy male baby.
- *At 25 years*: She delivered a stillborn male baby.
- *At 26 years*: She delivered a healthy female baby.
- *At 28 years*: She became pregnant, but it was terminated medically in first trimester.
- *At 30 years*: Her first child died of gastroenteritis.

Conclusion: The obstetric history of this female can be summarized as: "G7 P3 A3 L1 D2".

CHAPTER 14

Drug History

> *He is the best physician that knows the worthlessness of the most medicines.*
> —**Benjamin Franklin**

This section includes the information of medicines which are being taken by the patient for some other disease or purpose, if any. In some cases, this small information can prove itself valuable while planning the diagnosis and management of the disease of the patient. Following are few examples:

- The presenting complaints of a patient could be the adverse effect of some drug. For example:

> A young man presented with complaints of epigastric pain and hematemesis. He was a nonsmoker, nonalcoholic, and preferred nonspicy food, but his drug history revealed that he was taking some analgesics for backache since a month. It led his doctor to suspect drug-induced gastritis due to nonsteroidal anti-inflammatory drug (NSAID).

> A young woman presented with complaints of restlessness, involuntary movements, and uncontrolled speech. These were found to be extrapyramidal side effects of metoclopramide which she had taken for control of her hiccoughs.

> A young male presented with painless enlargement of both breasts (gynecomastia). It was found to be the side effect of ketoconazole which he was taking for the treatment of tinea capitis (fungal infection of scalp).

> A patient presented with complaints of nausea, vomiting, and jaundice. He was a known case of tuberculosis and was taking anti-tubercular treatment. This information helped the physician in suspecting isoniazid-induced hepatotoxicity in his case.

- If the patient is taking some drug for some other disease, it is essential for the physician to know about it while planning the treatment for his current disease. This information will help him in selecting the drugs which do not interact with other drugs being taken by the patient. For example:

> A young male presented with complaints of fever and sore throat to a physician. He made a diagnosis of pharyngitis and prescribed erythromycin for its treatment. Unfortunately, the patient was a known case of rheumatic heart disease and was taking warfarin since a year. Erythromycin increased the metabolism of warfarin which resulted in a fatal gastrointestinal bleeding.

> A gynecologist advised a young, married female to take oral contraceptive pills for contraception. She forgot to enquire about her drug history. The patient was taking anti-tubercular drugs for abdominal tuberculosis. Rifampicin increased the metabolism of steroids (of oral contraceptive pills) which resulted in a failure of contraception.

COMMONLY USED DRUGS

Following are some of the examples of medicines which are commonly used by the patients for various common diseases:
- *Antihypertensives, oral hypoglycemics, and insulin:* Especially by elderly patients suffering from hypertension and diabetes.
- *Antiepileptics:* By epilepsy patients.
- *Steroids and other drugs:* For the treatment of asthma.
- *Analgesics:* For arthritis, backache, etc.
- *Calcium supplements:* For osteoporosis in old age.
- *Oral contraceptive pills:* By women of reproductive age.
- *Homeopathic, Ayurvedic, Herbal or Unani medicines:* For various chronic diseases.

DRUGS FOR THE SAME DISEASE

Apart from knowing about the drugs for any other disease, it is important for a physician to know about the drugs which patient has taken for the same disease in the previous few days. This information

may be valuable for a physician for estimating the severity of disease and for planning its treatment. Following are few examples:
- If a patient is already taking some treatment for his disease, but is not getting any relief, physician can start some new treatment only if he knows about the previous one.

> A patient presented with features of mild reflux esophagitis. The physician was planning to start with some H2 receptor blocker (such as Ranitidine). But he found that the patient had already taken it on prescription of some other doctor, which did not bring any significant relief to him. So, he preferred to start with a drug from some different category, e.g., proton pump inhibitor.

> Respiratory infection of a child was not relieved by Cefadroxil (first generation cephalosporin) which was prescribed by his family physician. So, his pediatrician preferred to switch over to some other antibiotic and prescribed him Cefpodoxime (third generation cephalosporin), which effectively cured his illness.

- Self medication of some basic drugs (such as analgesics and antipyretics) is a common phenomenon. Severity of the signs and symptoms of any illness may get modified if the patient has already taken some treatment for his disease. For example:

> A patient, who had presented with complaints of high-grade fever and chills, was only mildly febrile on presentation. It was found to be due the effect of paracetamol which he had taken at his home, just a few hours before consulting his physician.

> A patient presented to an orthopedician with a history of recent traumatic injury to his right thumb. On clinical examination, he noticed mild local tenderness and suspected some minor injury only. But, he was surprised to see a fracture of proximal phalanx in his X-ray. This was because the patient had already taken some strong analgesic, few hours before consulting the orthopedician.

It is important for any physician to obtain the maximum possible information of the drugs being taken by the patient for his disease. Old documents are valuable but may not always available. Patient may not be able to recall the chemical name or brand name of the drug. Physician can get some clue by asking about the form (tablet/capsule/syrup), color, frequency, etc., of the drug. For example, a patient said that for his pain, he was taking a *pink colored large tablet* for three times in a day with milk. This information is pointing toward the possibility of *Brufen*, a popular brand of Ibuprofen.

A peculiar difficulty is encountered when some patient gives a history of taking some OTC (Over the counter) drugs for his problems. These are the drugs which are sold by the retailers at medical shops to their customers without any specific prescription. Common examples are antipyretics, analgesics, antacids, antiemetics, antidiarrheals, antibiotics, etc. Irrational indication and improper dosage are the common problems associated with OTC drugs, especially in the pediatric age groups.

CHAPTER 15

Allergy History

A doctor who cannot take a good history and a patient who cannot give one are in danger of giving and receiving bad treatment.
—Anonymous

Allergy is a hypersensitivity disorder of immune system. Allergic reactions occur when a person's immune system reacts abnormally to certain harmless substances, such as food, pollens, dust, drug, etc.

This section enquires about the history of any major or minor allergic reaction to any drug in the past life of the patient. This information is not much important in making the diagnosis of disease, but is more important for planning its management.

Drug allergy is an unpleasant and unpredictable phenomenon. A patient, who had well-tolerated a drug in past, may become allergic to it on subsequent exposure and vice versa.

Same drug may give different allergic manifestations in different individuals. Severity of allergic reactions ranges from mild itching to severe anaphylaxis and even death. Commonly seen allergic reactions are skin rashes, itching, urticaria, bronchospasm, allergic rhinitis, etc.

Some drugs which are well-known for their allergic potential are penicillin, sulfonamides, lignocaine, etc.

It is always better to be safe than sorry. It is essential for a physician to know about the allergic reaction to some drug in the past, if any. It will help him during planning the management of patient's present disease.

If a patient has suffered from some unpleasant reaction to any drug in past, he will remember it forever, but he may forget to mention about it unless he has been specifically asked by the doctor. So, history of any allergic reaction should be asked to each and every patient regardless of his presenting complaints.

> After his ophthalmic examination, an old man developed complaints of itching and burning sensation in his eyes. It was suspected that he was allergic to the eye drops containing phenylephrine, which were used for dilatation of his pupils. After few years, he visited some other ophthalmologist for his eye checkup. The doctor *forgot to ask* and the old man *forgot to inform* about history of any allergic reaction in past. Same drug was used for pupillary dilatation, which resulted in severe edema and congestion of his eyes.

Most of the patients understand about the allergic reaction when been asked as any "history of *allergy* or *reaction* to any medicine in past". Others can be asked by enquiring about the common symptoms of allergic reaction, such as—*did you ever suffer from any skin rash or itching or any other unpleasant effect after taking some drug?*

Whenever found positive, maximum possible enquiry should be done by the physician to know about the drug and the reaction caused by it. Allergic reaction to any drug is an unforgettable event and even the illiterate sufferers usually remember the name of the drug which had caused some unpleasant reaction in the past.

Occasionally, some patients wrongly use the word allergy for any major side effect caused by some drug in the past. An unpleasant response to any drug is not always some allergic reaction. Many time, it may be merely a side effect of that drug. For example, if a patient says that he had nausea and vomiting after taking some analgesic in past, it seems more likely to be the side effect of the drug rather than any allergic reaction. Nausea and vomiting are common side effects of many drugs and interestingly, many patients call such drugs as *hot medicines* or *heavy dose* of medicine. They erroneously start feeling that they are allergic to the drug.

Whenever there is a suspicion of any allergic reaction in the past, extreme precaution should be kept while prescribing the treatment for the current disease of the patient. The suspected drug and its congeners should be avoided and preference should be given to safer alternatives. If very much required, the suspected drug should be used with extreme precaution, preferably after ruling out any allergic reaction by appropriate investigations.

CHAPTER 16

Case History of Pediatric Patients

The way we talk to our children becomes their inner voice
—Peggy O'Mara

History taking in case of a pediatric patient needs some modifications in the general format, as it requires more emphasis on some additional information about the child. At the same time, many other points from general format are of little or no use for pediatric patients.

According to Indian Academy of Pediatrics (IAP), the spectrum of "pediatrics" ranges *from the birth to 18 years* of life. This period is further subdivided as:

- Newborn (Neonate) : First 4 weeks after birth
- Infant : First year
- Toddler : 1–3 years
- Preschool child : 3–6 years
- School-age child : 6–10 years (boys)
  6–12 years (girls)
- Adolescent : 10–18 years

FORMAT FOR PEDIATRIC HISTORY

1. Patient's profile
2. Presenting complaints
3. History of presenting complaints
4. Past history
5. Antenatal history
6. Birth history
7. Neonatal history
8. Developmental history
9. Dietary history
10. Immunization history
11. Family history
12. Contact history

13. Allergy history

Following is the detailed description of individual sections:

Patient's Profile

- *Name:* Name of a child should be mentioned along with his/her father's name and surname.

  For example: "Master Shreyas s/o Karan Singh Chauhan", "Baby Afreen d/o Javed Hussain," etc.

  Sometimes, parents may tell only the pet name of their child, e.g., Chunnu, Duggu, etc. If so, his/her real name (official name, i.e., name in records such as birth certificate/school, etc.) should be to be asked for his case history.

  If the child is yet to be named (e.g., newborn or young infant), he/she should be addressed by his mother's (preferably) or father's name as: "Baby of Padma Solanki", "Baby of Balvinder Kaur", etc.

- *Age:* During history taking, try to mention the age of a child up to most accurate extent. The unit of age depends upon the age group to which the child belongs. If possible, even the date of birth of all small children should be noted in case history.
  - Newborns: In days (e.g., 8 days old, 25 days old)
  - Infants: In months (e.g., 4 months old, 9 and half months old)
  - Toddlers: In years and months (e.g., 2 years and 4 months old)
  - Older children and adolescent: In years (e.g., 9 years, 15 years)

- *Sex:* The only condition in which one needs to ask about the sex of the patient is when he/she is a newborn or an infant.

  Many a time, gender of the child may be difficult to decide even from his/her name, e.g., unisex names, such as *Suman, Gurdeep, Kiran, Chandan,* etc.

  Occasionally, it is difficult to decide the gender of some old children only from their attire and appearance. For example, a female child may come dressed up in shorts and a T-shirt, which may make her look like a boy. Similarly, a male baby may be seen with his hair tied in a pony knot, which makes him look like a girl. Obviously, the problems related to internal and external genital organs will be exclusively seen in the children of corresponding sex only (e.g., phimosis, undescended testis, etc., in male children and synechia vulvae, ovarian cyst, etc., in female children). Apart from these, manifestation of some genetic disorders depends upon the sex of the child. For example, X-linked recessive diseases (e.g., hemophilia, red green color blindness) are more likely to occur in males than females (as males have only one X chromosome, defective gene is guaranteed to manifest in any male who carries it. While females have two X chromosomes. So, the chances of having two defective copies of the gene are remote in females, and they are almost exclusively the asymptomatic carriers of the disorder).

- *Residence:* Problems, such as worm infestation, scabies, tuberculosis, etc., are more commonly seen in children from slums and backward areas of the city. Respiratory problems in children may be due to allergy to pollution (in industrial area) or pollens (in rural area). This information also gives some clue for diagnosis of the diseases which are endemic to some districts and states (e.g., filariasis in Bihar, Orissa, etc.)
- *Religion:* Some diseases are more prevalent among people of a particular religion (sickle cell anemia in tribal and aboriginal population, thalassemia in Sindhis, Punjabis, etc.).
- *Occupation:* Except for the adolescent from low socioeconomic class, children are usually not involved in any occupational activity. Hence, this point is of little use for pediatric patients and may be replaced by *literacy* (i.e., information of educational status of child). For example, he is a student of 5th standard.

  However, occupation of one or both parents should be recorded, as it will be required to assess the socioeconomic status of the family. Also, in some cases, occupation of parents may lead to some risk of occupational hazards to their children as well. For example, features of lead poisoning may be seen in children of people involved in occupation of printing, battery manufacturing, etc. Parents who are exposed to lead in their workplace can bring lead dust home on skin or clothes, which leads to an exposure of their children also.

  Additionally, it is important to ask about scholastic performance of the child (can be described as average, above or below average), as it may get affected by current illness, e.g., chronic illness, such as sickle cell anemia, thalassemia, poorly controlled asthma, etc.
- *Socioeconomic status:* It should be assessed on the basis of per capita income of the family, type of house, number of rooms, sanitation, etc. Communicable diseases such as tuberculosis, worm infestation, etc., are more commonly seen in children from low socioeconomic class.

Presenting Complaints

In case of young children, most of the information is gained from their parents and grandparents. Name and relation of the person who is giving the details of child's illness should be mentioned as the "*Informant*" (e.g., mother, father, grandmother, etc.). In most of the cases, mother is the best and the most reliable source of information about the child. So, for any enquiry, she should be preferred over the others.

In case of neonates and young children, many symptoms are perceived by parents and pediatricians on basis of some indirect evidences. Few examples are:
- *Excessive cry:* For pain, hunger, thirst, wetting, fear, anxiety, local hurt
- *Refusal to feed:* For loss of appetite or any systemic illness causing reduced appetite
- *Crying and pulling of penis during micturition:* For burning sensation

Complaints should be presented according to the acts, and not as some interpretations. For example, it will be better to present as a complaint of "excessive crying and pulling of penis during micturition", rather than as "burning sensation in micturition".

Many parents present the problem of their child in an exaggerated form, especially if they are of over-caring nature. Most of such complaints are related to his diet or weight, such as "*he is not eating properly*", "*he has become very weak*", "*he is not gaining proper weight*". Some of these complaints may not have relation with actual disease of child. An experienced pediatrician knows this fact. But sometimes, an inexperienced student may overestimate the significance of these complaints. For example:

> A 5-year-old child was having a painless scrotal swelling for 3 months. On examination, it was found to be fluctuant, nontender, and brilliantly transilluminant, which was favoring toward a diagnosis of *hydrocele*. While a student was taking his history, her mother complained that her child had become *very weak* and was *not eating much* since he had developed that swelling. This information confused the student, as he could not correlate the complaints of weakness and anorexia with the diagnosis of hydrocele. In fact, he started thinking about some unrelated conditions, such as tuberculosis or malignancy.

History of Presenting Complaints

In this section, detailed enquiry should be made about the onset and features of symptoms and of course of the disease, as described in previous chapter on history of presenting complaints.

In general, history of presenting complaints of any patient begins from the time when he was not having the presenting symptoms (such as—*"My patient was apparently alright till two months back, when he noticed a small swelling on right side of his neck."*). But, history of a child who is *born with some congenital anomaly* should be presented in a different way.—*"As per mother of the child, he was born with a swelling at his lower back region."*

Past History

The contents of this section depend upon the age of the child. In a neonate or infant, it is desirable to know about any significant event *during or before his birth* (which is included in a separate section of "birth and antenatal history"). But the same information may or may not be of much significance for older children and adolescents. In their case, it will be more significant to enquire about the history of any of common childhood illnesses in their past life, such as:

- *History of diseases, such as:* Tuberculosis (TB), measles (*Khasra*), mumps (*Gal-sua*), whooping cough (*Kali khaansi, Kukkar khaansi*), hepatitis, jaundice (*Peeliya*), chickenpox (*Chhoti mata, Masoori, Chhoti chechak*), etc.
- History of hospitalization
- History of blood transfusion (in cases of hemolytic disorders such as thalassemia, sickle cell anemia, etc.)
- History of any surgery
- History of similar complaints in past
- In cases of neurological problems, such as encephalitis, history of *animal bites* or of *recent vaccination* should be asked.

Antenatal History

This part is more significant for neonates and infants, but should be extended for children up to 5 years of age. It includes information about any significant event during pregnancy or in the puerperium of the mother. Any kind of intrauterine exposure (mentioned later) to the developing fetus may manifest in the form of some disease in his later life. Following questions should be asked from the mother:

- Did you undergo regular antenatal checkups during pregnancy?
  A major cause of increased incidence of adverse outcomes of pregnancy [e.g., prematurity, low birth weight (LBW), congenital anomalies] in low socioeconomic class females is the lack of proper medical checkups during antenatal period.
- Were you immunized during pregnancy?
  Two doses of tetanus toxoid during pregnancy reduce the risk of neonatal tetanus.
- Whether the antenatal sonography was performed regularly? If yes, was there anything abnormal detected? (e.g., fetal maturity, amount of liquor, any congenital anomaly, etc.)
- Did you receive any medicines/supplements during pregnancy? (e.g., iron and folic acid tablets, medicines for thyroid, any other hormonal pills, antiepileptic drugs, etc.)
  - Chances of neural tube defects (e.g., meningocele, etc.) increases in fetus, if mother is suffering from folic acid deficiency.
  - Deficiency of iron: Anemia in pregnancy may lead to preterm delivery and LBW baby.
- Did you receive adequate nutrition during pregnancy?
  One extra meal with a balanced diet is recommended during pregnancy.
- Did you suffer from any significant problem (e.g., hypertension, diabetes, jaundice, etc.) during pregnancy?
  - Pregnancy-induced hypertension (PIH) may lead to a premature labor and LBW baby.
  - Maternal diabetes may lead to complications such as large for date (LFD) baby, hypocalcemia, etc.
  - History of TORCH infection may be suggested by history of unexplained fever with rashes in antenatal period.
  - History of swelling over body (for pre-eclampsia) and seizures (for eclampsia) during pregnancy.
  - History of any abnormal leaking, bleeding per vaginum, threatened abortion, etc. during pregnancy.
- Had you taken any drugs, especially in first trimester of pregnancy?
  Few examples of drugs with teratogenic potential are:
  - Valproic acid   : Neural tube defect
  - Streptomycin   : Deafness
  - Phenytoin   : Cleft lip, cleft palate
  - Antithyroid drugs   : Neonatal hypothyroidism

- Did you get any radiation exposure (e.g., X-ray), especially in the first trimester of pregnancy?
  - Radiation exposure in pregnancy may lead to complications such as growth retardation, mental retardation, etc. of the child.

Birth History

This is an enquiry about the information related to the birth of the child and the period immediately after it. It includes:
- What was the gestational age of child at the time of birth? Whether he was born full term (completed 37 weeks) or preterm?
  In some cases, when mother and other family members are unable to reply confidently, expected date of delivery (EDD) can be calculated from the last menstrual period (LMP) of the mother as:

  EDD = First day of LMP + 9 months and 7 days

  Problems, such as neonatal sepsis, developmental delay, undescended testis, congenital anomalies, etc., are more common in cases of prematurely delivered babies.
- Where was the delivery conducted? Whether at hospital or at home?
  This question is of more significance in cases of rural and low socio-economic class patients, as cases of home delivery are extremely rare in middle and upper class population, especially from urban areas. Problems, such as birth asphyxia, neonatal sepsis, etc., are more frequently seen in home delivered babies, even if the delivery was conducted by a trained birth attendant (*Dai*).
- What was the mode of delivery? Whether vaginal or cesarean?
  Usually, words such as *normal* and *operation* are used for vaginal and cesarean deliveries, respectively, even by rural and uneducated persons. In case of vaginal delivery, an enquiry should be made that whether instruments such as Forceps (*Auzaar*) or some minor procedure, such as episiotomy (*Cheera*) were required at the time of delivery. Episiotomy is a surgically planned incision on the perineum and posterior vaginal wall during second stage of labor. If mother gives history of use of some incision during delivery, it indicates toward episiotomy and should not be confused with cesarean section.

In routine practice, this part of birth history in recorded as acronyms such as *FTND at home* [full term, normal (vaginal) delivery at home] or *preterm LSCS D at hospital* (preterm, lower segment cesarean section delivery at hospital)

- If the baby was delivered by cesarean section, what was the indication?
  Cesarean section is recommended when vaginal delivery might pose some risk to mother or baby. Fetal distress, cord loop around neck, abnormal presentation (e.g., transverse lie, breech), meconium-stained liquor, etc., are some of the common indications for cesarean section.
- Whether the child had cried immediately after birth?
  This is to rule out the possibility of birth asphyxia. For example, in case of a 5-year-old child with delayed developmental milestones, the mother informs that he did not cry immediately after birth. Chances of hypoxic damage to brain (secondary to birth asphyxia) are likely to have occurred in this case.
- What was the birth weight of baby?
  In our country, average birth weight of a full-term neonate is approximately 2.8 kg, while less than 2.5 kg is considerd as low birth weight (LBW). Problems, such as neonatal sepsis, hypothermia, necrotizing enterocolitis, etc., are more common in LBW babies.
  This information is unavailable in most cases of home delivered babies, as no proper instrument is available at homes to measure the weight of a newborn. In many cases, weight of the child is recorded for the first time in an *anganwadi* after some days of his birth, which is usually different from the actual birth weight (because of physiological loss and regaining of body weight in first few days of life).
  Some parents may mention the birth weight in unit of *pounds*. One pound is equivalent to approximately 450 g. So, if parents say that child's birth weight was 6 pounds, it will be approximately 2.7 kg.

Neonatal History

Duration from birth to first 28 days of life is known as the neonatal period. This is one of the most significant phases of life when a child has to adapt himself to the external environment. Following are some of the important queries to be enquired about this period:
- Did he develop jaundice in the neonatal period? If yes, then what was its pattern?

About 70% of neonates develop jaundice on second or third day of life (physiological jaundice) which lasts for about 5 days (in full-term babies) to 7 days (in preterm babies). Any deviation from this normal pattern of appearance and disappearance points toward some abnormality and is known as pathological jaundice. Rh incompatibility, ABO incompatibility, neonatal sepsis, etc., are some of the important causes of pathological jaundice in neonates.

- When did he pass urine and meconium?
  Most of the neonates pass meconium within 24 hours and urine within 48 hours. Delayed passage of meconium may be seen in case of Hirschsprung's disease, infants of diabetic mothers, etc. Similarly, delayed passage of urine may be an indication of an underlying congenital urologic anomaly.
- Was he hospitalized in the neonatal period?
  Admission in neonatal intensive care unit (NICU) may be required for some serious conditions, such as birth asphyxia, meconium aspiration, neonatal sepsis, neonatal jaundice, etc. Some parents give this history as that their child was kept in a glass box (*kaanch ki peti*) or under blue light (for phototherapy).
- When did his umbilical cord fall off?
  Umbilical cord is commonly known by various names, such as *naal, naadi,* etc. Mostly, it falls from 7–10 days after birth (range: 3–45 days). Delayed separation of umbilical cord may be seen in case of preterm babies and neonatal sepsis. In cases of home delivery, an enquiry should be made about the material used to cut and tie the umbilical cord. Improper cutting of umbilical cord may lead to infection of stump and umbilical sepsis.
- Any other significant problem in neonatal period?
  Parents should be asked about history of any other problem such as feeding difficulty, respiratory distress, seizures, etc., in neonatal period of child.

Developmental History

Development of a child refers to the biological, psychological, and emotional changes that occur in human beings between birth and the end of adolescence. This section of pediatric history enquires about the sequence and time of achievement of various developmental milestones of the child.

Section 3: Format of Medical History

Developmental milestones are a set of functional skills or age-specific tasks that most children are able to perform after a certain age range. Broadly, they can be divided in four categories:
1. Gross motor development
2. Fine motor and adaptive development
3. Personal social development
4. Language development

Following are some examples of commonly enquired developmental milestones, along with the age at which most of the children attain them. Complete list of all the milestones can be obtained from any standard textbook of pediatrics.

1. Gross motor
   a. Neck holding : 3 months
   b. Sitting without support : 8 months
   c. Crawling : 9 months
   d. Standing without support : 12 months
   e. Walking without support : 13 months
   f. Running : 18 months
2. Fine motor and adaptive
   a. Grasps objects placed in hands : 4 months
   b. Bidextrous grasp : 5 months
   c. Palmar grasp : 7 months
   d. Pincer grasp : 9 months
3. Personal social development
   a. Social smile : 2 months
   b. Recognizes mother : 3 months
   c. Smiles at mirror image : 6 months
   d. Waves "bye-bye" : 9 months
4. Language development
   a. Turns head to the sound : 1 month
   b. Cooing : 3 months
   c. Monosyllables ("ma", "ba") : 6 months
   d. Bisyllables ("mama", "baba") : 9 months
   e. Simple sentence : 24 months

The age mentioned along with each milestone is the age at which most of the children achieve it. In fact, it can be considered as the mean of age range, as few children achieve it a little earlier, while few others may attain it little late. In other words, the pace of development varies from child to child. For example, walking without support is attained by most of the children by 13th month. But, it is not unusual to find children who achieve this milestone at a younger age. At the same time, if a child starts walking without support at 13½ months, it should not be straightway considered as a case of delayed development.

If parents are unable to recall the exact age of their child at the time of achievement of a particular milestone, they may be simply asked to compare the child's development with the development of his elder siblings, if any.

Female children usually achieve these milestones little earlier than the male children. Also, even a normal child may miss some milestone such as crawling; he may start walking directly.

Dietary History

The questionnaire of the dietary history depends upon the age of the patient, as there is a significant difference in the diet of an infant and a grown up child. So, the questions should be problem oriented as well as age dependent. The common questions to be asked in this section are:

- Is the baby on breast milk or top feed?
  Breast milk is called by mother by various names such as *Maa ka doodh, Aang ka doodh, Chhati ka doodh,* etc. Other words, such as *Upar ka doodh* is used for the milk other than breast milk (e.g., cow milk, etc.), *Dabbe ka doodh* for formula milk, and *Upar ka khan*a for solid food (e.g., daliya, khichadi, etc.).
- If he is on breast milk, is he receiving it in sufficient amount, i.e., to his satiety?
  This is indicated by sound sleep after feeding, adequate urination, and weight gain.
- If he is not on breastfeeding, what is the reason? (e.g., lactational failure, unavailability/illness of mother, etc.)
- If he is on top feed, what is it: cow's milk or formula milk? What is the amount and frequency of feeding?
  Goat's milk is particularly deficient in folic acid, which may lead to megaloblastic anemia.
- If he is on cow's milk, is it diluted or undiluted? Does mother add sugar to it? If yes, how much sugar is added?
- If he is on formula milk, which formula is being used? (Preterm formula milk or term formula milk).
- If his weaning has been started, what was the age at which semisolid and solid food were introduced? What are the different solid foods given to him?
- What is the proportion of fiber in his total diet? (e.g., green vegetables, fruits, whole grain cereals, legumes, etc.)

- Is there any problem associated with any specific solid food? e.g., wheat (celiac disease, wheat allergy), milk (lactose intolerance) or egg (egg allergy), etc.?

Normally, in the first few months of life, an infant is exclusively on breastfeeding, which is gradually weaned and semi-solid food is introduced. Although, breastfeeding can be continued up to 2 years, gradual introduction of supplementary food should be started after 6 months of life. But, it is erroneously continued for prolonged periods (even up to 4–5 years) by some mothers, especially of low socio-economic class. This gives rise to problems, such as iron deficiency anemia, malnutrition, constipation, etc.

Infants who are on top feed are at a higher risk of suffering from gastroenteritis, malnutrition, etc., as compared to the infants who are on breast milk.

Constipation is more common in children who consume a large amount of nonfiber diet. Commonly consumed nonfiber diets by children of our country are biscuits, *tosh, gaanthiya* (namkeen), bread, pasta, noodles, etc. In general, most of these edible items are prepared from *Maida* (the refined wheat flour) or *Besan* (cereal flour made from ground chickpeas).

Immunization History

Incomplete immunization of children is still a commonly encountered problem in our country. It is not unusual to find a child who has missed few or all of his vaccines. So, an enquiry should be made about the immunization status of every child, regardless of the disease with which he has presented (immunization schedule recommended by the Indian Academy of Pediatrics can be obtained from any standard textbook of pediatrics).

No doubt that for this information, nothing will be better than the immunization card of the child. But unfortunately, it may not be available in many cases. Parents may not be able to remember the name of various vaccines. In such situation, some information can be drawn from the *site* of vaccination and *age* of the child at the time of immunization. For example:
- *BCG vaccine:* At the time of/shortly after birth, on left shoulder. Presence of scar of BCG vaccine confirms vaccination, but its absence does not.
- *Oral polio vaccine:* Given per orally, in form of drops.

- *DPT vaccine:* 1½, 2½, 3½ months, booster doses at 18 months and 5 years, on lateral aspect of thigh. It is usually associated with fever and swelling at the site of vaccination.
- *MR/MMR vaccine:* 9 months, on arm/forearm.

Family History

Under this section, enquiry should be made about:
- Health details of all family members (about their age, sex, any past or present illness, etc.).
- History of similar illness to any other sibling (it is important in cases of genetically transmitted diseases as well as contagious diseases).
- Age of mother at the time of delivery.
  Young age (<18 years) is associated with increased chances of preterm and IUGR babies while advanced age (>32 years) is associated with increased incidence of disorders such as Down syndrome.
  Advanced age of father is associated with an increased risk of Marfan's syndrome in the child.
- History of abortions or stillbirths.
  Some conditions such as chromosomal anomalies, maternal syphilis, etc., are associated with increased incidence of abortion and stillbirths.
- History of birth of an abnormal child in the family.
- History of death of any sibling. If occurred, then what was the cause of death?
- Special cases:
  - History of consanguineous marriage: Consanguineous marriage is the marriage solemnized among the persons who have descended from a common ancestor, i.e., are in close relation with each other. Probability of expression of autosomal recessive disorders increases in children born by such marriages (e.g., cystic fibrosis, thalassemia, sickle cell anemia, etc.).
  - Adopted child: Rarely, if the child is found to be adopted by his parents, this information should be mentioned specifically in this section. In cases of hereditary diseases, it would be essential to know about the health status of the biological parents, and not of the adoptive parents of the child.

Contact History

This is more significant in case of communicable diseases (e.g., tuberculosis, gastroenteritis, worm infestation, hepatitis A, typhoid, scabies, respiratory infections, etc.). These diseases spread by various modes such as physical contact, aerosols, feco-oral route, etc. Source of infection may be a family member, a neighbor, or some classmate, etc.

Allergy History

An enquiry should be made if child is allergic to any medicine (as described in general format) or food (e.g., wheat, cow's milk, peanuts, egg, etc.).

Section 4

Student–Patient Interaction

Section Outline

- How to Take and Present a Case History?
- An Illustrated Case History

CHAPTER 17

How to Take and Present a Case History?

You cannot truly listen to anyone and do anything else at the same time.

—*Scott Peck*

Student life is a brief but important phase of any doctor's life. During this period, he learns about the art of communication with different types of the patients. In every medical college hospital, a patient comes in contact with a consultant as well as the medical students. Both of them interact with him, but there is a significant difference in their communication with the same patient. Following **Table 17.1** shows some of the salient differences between history taking by a medical student and by a consultant or medical practitioner.

TABLE 17.1: Differences between history taking by a medical student and a medical practitioner.

Medical student	*Medical practitioner*
■ A medical student is in the learning phase of his life and "history taking" is an important part of his medical education	A medical practitioner is a learned physician. He is in professional phase of his life and his primary aim is to cure his patients
■ Mostly, he has to interrogate the patients who are admitted in the ward of a hospital (i.e., he is not the first medical person who interacts with the patient). Patients may not take him seriously, unless he is very confident while interacting with them	He mostly gets the patients in his outpatient department (OPD) or casualty (i.e., mostly, he is the first medical person who interacts with the patient). Patients put more faith in him, mainly due to his age and designation
■ He has to take a systematic and detailed history (including all questions from the standard format) of the patient and examine him thoroughly	He is not bound to ask all questions of the format. He mainly focuses on the relevant questions and examination, depending upon the disease of the patient

Contd...

Contd...

Medical student	Medical practitioner
■ He usually gets a limited time (e.g., 30 minutes) for history taking and examination of the patient	He is not bounded by any time limit. But still, he does not spend excessively long time in interrogation and examination of the patients, as he has to see multiple patients in a short duration
■ He mostly interacts with stable patients with chronic complaints. Patients with acute problems (e.g., myocardial infarction, perforation peritonitis, trauma patients, etc.) are not suitable for interaction with undergraduate students	He has to deal with acute as well as chronic patients, depending upon his field of specialization
■ After noting down all the details, he has to present his case history to his teacher or examiner	He does not have to present his history to any other person
■ His task is mainly to make a clinical diagnosis of patient's disease. Beyond that, he cannot decide or change the line of management of the patient. Still, he is expected to have a theoretical knowledge of further investigations and treatment of the patient	He takes the history of the patient to make a clinical diagnosis. After that, he sends the patient for some investigations (if required) and then prescribes the suitable treatment for his disease
■ Because of having only superficial knowledge and little practical experience of different diseases, it is difficult for a student to confidently judge the relative significance of different information provided by the patient. So, during student life, he should *ask all the questions* (of standard format), *listen to everything*, and *record almost everything* for presentation	A practicing doctor has got a better theoretical knowledge and practical experience of different diseases. So, he is able to segregate the information given by the patients on basis of their significance. Hence, during his practice, he asks only the significant questions, listens to everything, but records only the relevant information
■ If a student makes some mistake in his task, it will only lead to some loss of his academic impression or of his marks in examinations	A mistake done by a medical practitioner may lead to a wrong diagnosis and an improper treatment, which may even endanger the life of the patient

SUFFERINGS OF A PATIENT

Before communicating with any patient, every student should be aware of following facts and precautions:
- Never presume that history taking is your right and it is the responsibility of every patient to allow you for conversation and examination. Modesty and humbleness are essential to gain the confidence and cooperation of any patient.
- Your patient may have very poor knowledge and intelligence. Understand his limitations and be cooperative in your communication. Do not get annoyed if he is unable to understand your questions properly. If your feel that it is difficult for you to reach his level, then remember that it is rather *impossible* for him to reach to your level.
- Your patient may be looking comfortable from his external appearance. But internally, he may be going through one of the most stressful phases of his life. Be gentle and empathetic toward him.

HISTORY TAKING

History taking is an art and every doctor improves it throughout his life, right from the beginning of his student life. Following are some suggestions for medical students to improve their communication with patients during clinical postings and practical examinations:

First Impression

Well said by someone that the first impression is the last impression. Before approaching any patient, you should be aware of your dressing and appearance. No patient will show a serious interest in talking to a young medical student with shabby beard, untidy clothes, or dirty apron. Hectic working life should not be an excuse, especially during internship and postgraduation. Even if your appearance is not ideal, it should not be objectionable at least (**Fig. 17.1**).

Proper Time and Place

The act of history taking and clinical examination needs significant time of student and patient. Make sure that your patient remains

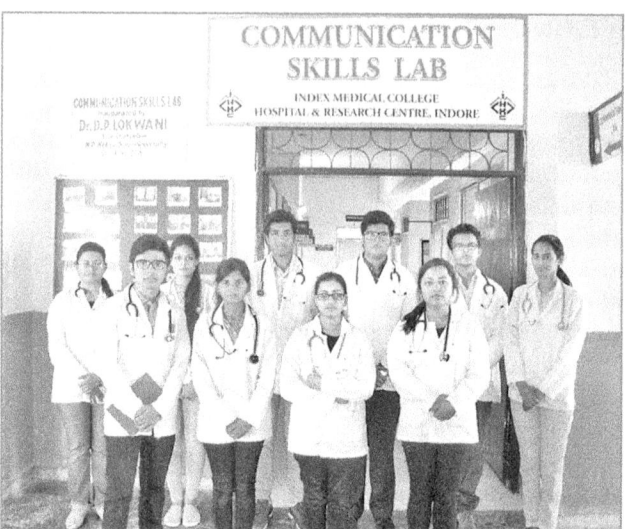

Fig. 17.1: Descent appearance suits medical profession.

comfortable throughout the process. Occasionally, you may find the patient in a situation which is unsuitable for proper communication. For example, a hungry patient who is about to start his lunch or a mother who is feeding her baby may not be able to converse comfortably. So, in such conditions, do not force your patient to communicate and cooperate with you. It would be better to postpone the conversation till the time he or she is well prepared for conversation.

Similarly, select the most comfortable place for communication with your patient. If you anticipate a significant interference from the chaos of other people in the ward, prefer to communicate with the patient at some isolated place, if possible.

Accompanying Person

If your patient is accompanying with some relative, ask about his or her relation with the patient. This information will help you in deciding the comfort and cooperation of your patient during communication. For example, a female with some gynecological problem will be most comfortable in conversing with you in front of her husband, but not in presence of some other male member of her family. So, before starting your conversation with your patient, make sure that he or

Chapter 17: How to Take and Present a Case History?

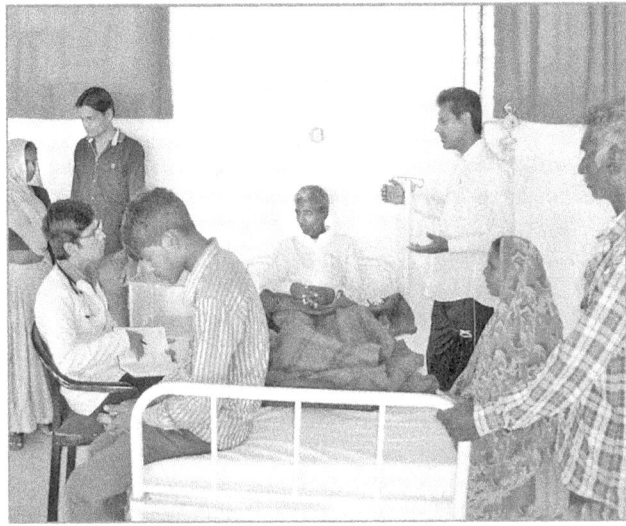

Fig. 17.2: Distraction in communication by surrounding persons.

she is comfortable for it in presence of the accompanying person. Sometimes, patient may prefer to call some other relative from outside the ward.

If you find that your patient is surrounded by a large number of relatives or visitors, gently request them to leave the patient for some time for conversation with you (**Fig. 17.2**). But at the same time, allow at least one or two close relatives to stay with the patient, as some patients feel quite uncomfortable in communicating with students or doctors in all alone, especially the female patients. Ideally, the selection of suitable relative should be left to the choice of the patient. In fact, in some cases, patient is unable to give proper history and so, presence of some close relative is essential to confirm or obtain the information, e.g., elderly or uncooperative patient.

The most reliable information about any disease can be provided by patient only. But sometimes, you may find some relative who is replying to your questions and not allowing the patient to answer them. This interference may annoy you after some time, especially if your patient is able to answer these questions of his own. Handle this situation calmly and ask the relative to let the patient reply first. Ensure him that you will take his help if the patient is unable to reply any question properly. This problem is more commonly seen in cases of adolescent and elderly patients.

Introduce Yourself

First of all, introduce yourself to the patient. Inform the patient that you are a medical student. Inform him that the senior doctor (the consultant) has sent you to ask about his disease and that you are going to tell the senior doctor about his problems. For example:

Namaskar. *Aap kaise hai? Mera naam Abhinav Saxena hai. Bade doctor sahib ne mujhe aapki takleef ke bare me aapse kuchh puchhne ke liye kaha hai, jo mai baad me unhe batane waala hu. Kya abhi aapse baat kar sakta hu?*

("Hello. How are you? My name is Abhinav Saxena. My senior doctor has asked me to have a talk with you about your disease. I will discuss with him about it later. Can we talk right now?").

This beginning will definitely increase the interest of the patient in having some conversation with you. He may feel that this conversation is definitely going to bring some benefit to his treatment and hence he will heartily cooperate with you during conversation and examination. In contrast, if you directly start taking the medical history, some patients may not take you seriously.

During clinical postings, do not visit your patient in a large group. He may get disturbed by a surprising visit of a large number of medical students. It will be better if you first choose a leading student from your batch. He or she should first visit to the patient to take his permission. Other students should join him, as soon as the conversation begins. The major interaction of patient should occur with the leading student only. Patient may get annoyed if he faces multiple questions from multiple students. Other students should silently observe this interaction (**Figs. 17.3 to 17.5**).

Avoid taking history in standing position. This may make you feel fatigued after sometime. Moreover, standing position of student will not be comfortable for the patient also because prolonged upward gaze (to make eye contact with a standing student) may make him uncomfortable after sometime. This discomfort may lead to a loss of his interest in conversation with the student (**Figs. 17.6 and 17.7**).

Use Appropriate Language

Proper selection of words is very important during communication with any person. Any kind of conversation will be unsuccessful if the spoken words are not understood by any of the member of dyad, i.e., doctor or patient. Remember the following points to know the

Chapter 17: How to Take and Present a Case History?

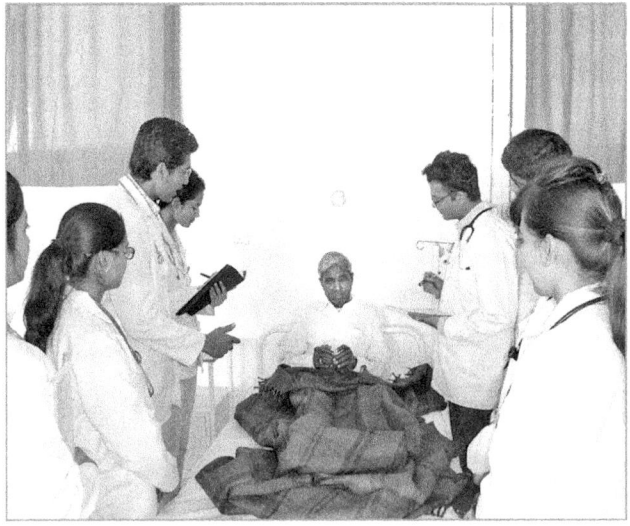

Fig. 17.3: Simultaneous questioning by multiple students.

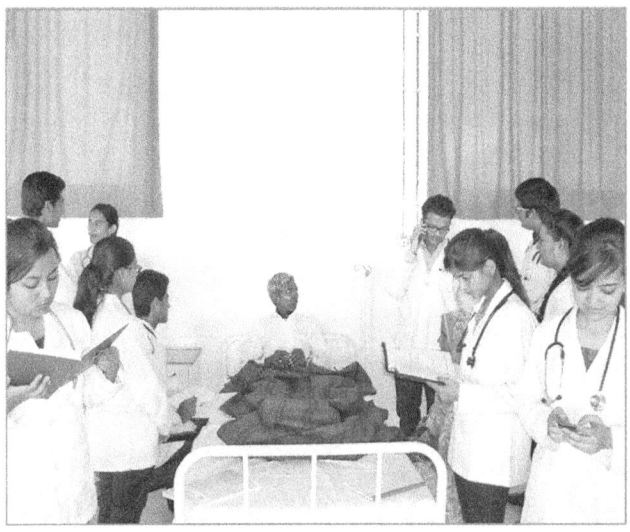

Fig. 17.4: Distraction in communication by students.

Section 4: Student–Patient Interaction

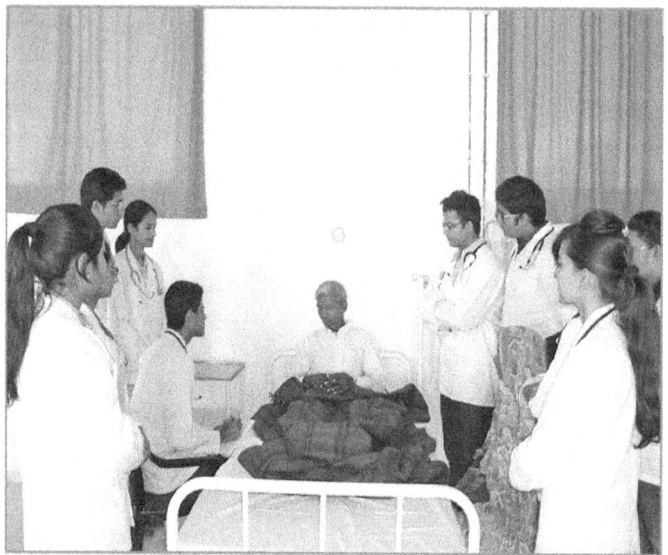

Fig. 17.5: Leading student with silent observers.

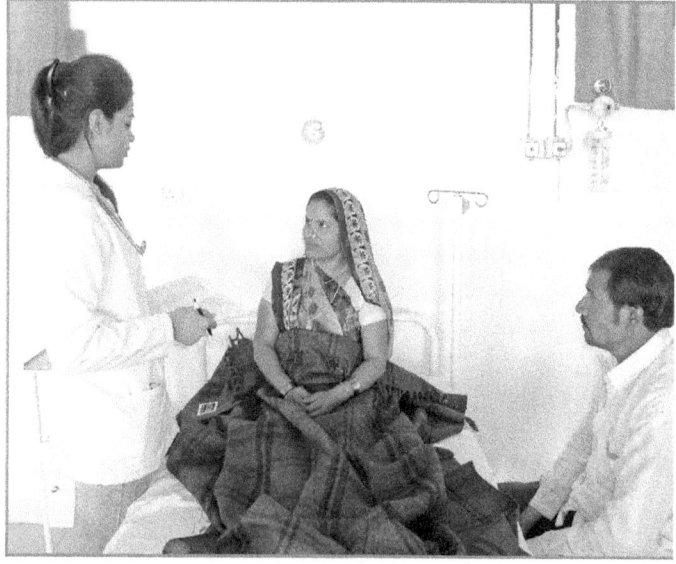

Fig. 17.6: Eyes of student and patient at different levels.

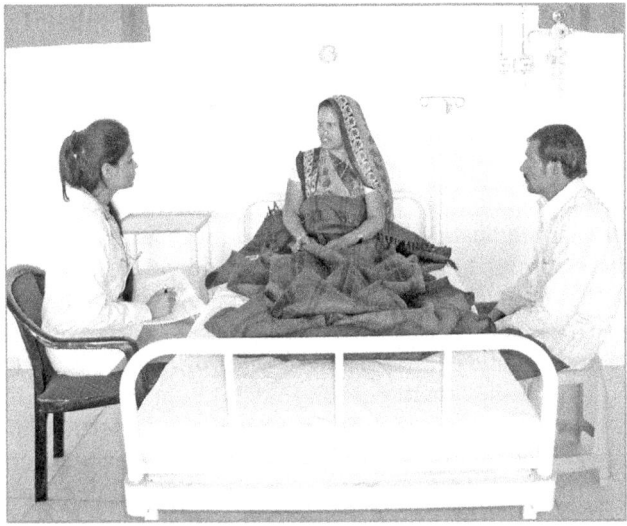

Fig. 17.7: Eyes at the same level.

importance of proper language during communication with your patients:
- Assess the preferred language and intellectual level of your patient during initial moments of conversation. Most of the patients are comfortable for conversation in Hindi or their regional language (such as Marathi, Gujarati, etc.) only.
- You can use the commonly spoken English words (such as sugar, allergy, toilet, etc.) only if you feel that your patient is intelligent enough to understand them. Otherwise, avoid using English words, and prefer the word which is better understood by your patient.
- Avoid using any medical terminology while taking history of any patient. Even the most intelligent and educated patients may not be able to understand some commonly spoken medical words, e.g., gastritis, colitis, malignancy, etc.
- Tailor your language according to the intellectual level of your patient. Same word may not be suitable for all types of patient. For example, if you have to ask about the history of diabetes, an illiterate person may find it difficult to understand if you ask him as *diabetes* and a well-educated person may feel offended if you ask him as *shakkar ki beemari*. A single question can be asked in multiple ways. The choice of appropriate words should be

done according to the understanding and intellectual level of the patient.
- If you feel that your patient is finding some difficulty in understanding some word, repeat your question with the suitable translation of that word.
- If you belong to some different state and are not well-versed with the regional language of your college (e.g., a student from south India in a medical college of some Hindi speaking state and vice versa), try your best to improve your knowledge of the regional language. Your friends could be of great help in this training. In the beginning and in extreme cases, you can take the help of some interpreter while communicating with your patient.
- Even in a single language, you may find patients with different dialects at different places. Dialect is a particular form of language which is peculiar to specific region or group. For example, *Avadhi, Chhattisgarhi, Malvi*, etc., are some of the dialects of Hindi language. It is well said for our country that here *water changes at every two miles and language changes at every four miles*. At present, there are 22 official languages in India and each of them includes different dialects. With frequent communication with your patients, you will find yourself more comfortable with conversing in the dialect of your place.
- Some words are commonly spoken and understood by the residents of a particular geographical area or community. Such words are more commonly used by rural, elderly, traditional, and urban poor people. For example, *safaai* for medical termination of pregnancy, *sikaai* for radiotherapy, *kala motiya* for glaucoma, *dhaat* for urethral discharge, etc. Whenever you come across any such new word, try to find its meaning from your colleagues, seniors, or teachers and prefer to use them during your subsequent conversation with such patients. This will definitely improve your understanding and communication with them. In contrast, lack of knowledge about these strange words may sometimes create a difficult situation, both for student and the patient. For example:

> After doing his graduation from Delhi, a student opted for postgraduation in surgery in a medical college of central India. He was taking history of a 45-year-old rural woman with a swelling in her neck. When he asked her about any surgery in her past life, she informed that she had undergone *bada operation* 5 years back.

> The literal meaning of bada operation is "big or major surgery". Naturally, he became curious to know about its details like duration of surgery, indication, etc. He got confused when she told him that it was done for excessive vaginal bleeding and was finished in just 1 hour. He was highly puzzled until his senior clarified him that she was talking about "hysterectomy". At many places of our country, hysterectomy and tubectomy are commonly known by the local people as *bada operation* and *chhota operation*, respectively.

- During your conversation, keep addressing your patient by his or her name (such as *Mr Joshi, Ramsingh ji, Varsha ji*, etc.) or some other appropriate words (such as *dada, amma, chacha, bhaiya, behenji*, etc.), depending upon his age and socioeconomic status. Frequent use of such words during conversation shows a feeling of empathy and caring attitude of student toward his patient.

Proper Nonverbal Communication

While taking history of your patient, you should look quite interested in knowing about his problem and confident and specific while asking your questions. This will give a positive impression to your patient and he would respond in the same way. Your body language plays a major role here. Remember the following suggestions:

- Make proper eye contact with your patient, both while asking any question and while listening to his answers. A good eye contact during speaking makes you look more confident in communication. Similarly, adequate eye contact during listening makes the other person feel that you are interested in the conversation.
- Keep nodding your head while listening to the patient, along with some vocal cues (sounds from vocal cords). This gives him a positive feedback that you are listening to his problems attentively. Also, this encourages him to speak more about his disease.
- Make appropriate conversational gestures by your hand, especially while asking or explaining some difficult question. This will make you look more confident and specific during conversation. Some hand gestures may help the patient to understand or reply the question in a better way. For example, clenching of fist for colicky pain, showing thumb and index finger for size of some swelling or ulcer, etc.

- Avoid listening to your patient with an expressionless mask-like face. The appropriate variation of facial expressions of the listener (such as happy, sad, surprised, etc.) gives a positive and pleasant feedback to the speaker. For example, if a patient informs you that an extremely large tumor was removed from his abdomen few years ago, he will be satisfied if he notices some expressions of surprise on your face.
- Converse with your patient in moderate volume. Most of the times, the student–patient communication occurs in an open ward. Your patient may not feel comfortable if his problems are being heard by the other patients of the ward. So, remember to keep your volume at moderate level. It should be further lowered down while asking some relatively personal questions, such as addiction, menstrual history, etc.
- Avoid writing while you are conversing with your patient, especially when he is telling you some important details of his problem, e.g., in section of history of presenting complaints. The act of writing obviously breaks your eye contact with the patient. So, it will be better if you first listen to his brief speech without any interruption. Start writing the important points in your history sheet only when he has finished speaking. If his history is long, before writing, it will be better to present its summary to the patient for his confirmation.

Avoid Checking the Documents

Do not check the case file or old documents of your patient, even if they are easily available to you. Do not try to find the diagnosis of your patient from any source and try your best to make a provisional diagnosis of your own. Continue this habit in your clinical practice also.

> During their clinical posting, a batch of undergraduate students was asked by the consultant to take history of a patient in medicine ward. Before visiting the patient, students came to know about his diagnosis as "mitral stenosis" from some postgraduate student. All of them read specifically about the clinical features and management of mitral stenosis from their books. Though the patient was not having the classical features of mitral stenosis, still the students were able to somehow extract his symptoms in favor of the same. It led to a bizarre presentation in front of the consultant as he was a case of *chronic bronchitis* with absolutely normal cardiac function. This error occurred because the postgraduate student had wrongly told them the diagnosis of some other case. Some students were even able to auscultate a diastolic murmur in his mitral area.

How to Write?

The standard format of medical history includes a number of sections and questions, which should be asked to the patient in a specific sequence. It is essential for every student to memorize all questions of the format, but it may be slightly difficult task in the beginning. Student may forget to ask some important question or may ask the questions in random sequence. Some other students try to recall some question in front of the patient, which obviously give him a negative impression about them. No doubt that this knowledge definitely improves with time and practice. But still, the beginners are suggested to practice it in a different way. If some student is not confident about his memory of questions, then even before meeting his patient, he should first write the headings of all sections and questions on his sheet (**Fig. 17.8**).

Even if you are taking patient's history on printed sheets of logbook, still you should memorize all questions of the format. Otherwise, you may find difficulty in recalling the questions when you have to take some patient's history on a blank sheet, e.g., during your practical examinations.

Practice to finish your task (of history taking and examination of patient) in a specified time. This habit will help you in your practical examinations, when you get only a limited period to do the same task.

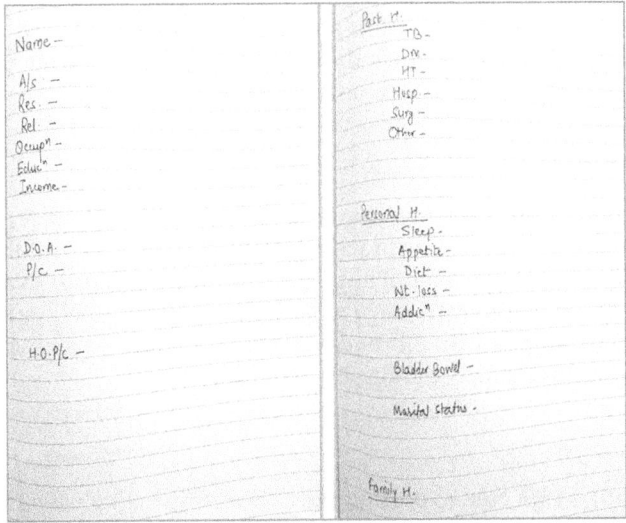

Fig. 17.8: A good method of recording case history for the beginners.

How to Conclude?

After finishing your task of history taking and examination, do not forget to thank the patient for providing you the information about his disease. Assure him that you will convey his information to senior consultant. Wish him a speedy recovery and healthy life. Also, whenever you visit the same ward again in next few days, do not forget to meet your patient again for few minutes. By doing so, you will learn about the progress of his treatment and he will be pleased by noticing your caring attitude.

▌PRESENTATION OF CASE HISTORY

Just like any food dish, presentation of a case history is as important as its preparation. If not presented properly, even a nicely cooked nutritious dish may be disliked by the people. Same problem can happen with a case history also.

The role of a medical student is of a communicator between the patient and his teacher or examiner. First, he interacts with the patient in a language which is easily understood by him. By doing do, he obtains various types of information from him. Then, he tailors them according to their significances and finally, he presents these information in front of his teacher or examiner in a systematic order in English language.

The skill of presentation of case history can only be improved by regular practice. Following are some important suggestions for medical students to improve their presentation skill during clinical postings and practical examinations:

First Impression

First impression is the last impression. On the day of presentation during clinical posting or practical examinations, be careful about your dressing and personal appearance. Your teacher or examiner may take any such negligence negatively. Similarly, make sure that you are possessed with all required materials, such as stethoscope, torch, measuring tape, percussion hammer, etc.

Language

A student is expected to present the case history in English language. During presentation, any grammatical or pronunciation mistake may give a negative impression to the listener. Please do not get discouraged if you are not having a good command on English language because a good examiner will first assess your knowledge of medical science and not of spoken English. Still, you should try your best to improve the command on your language by making multiple presentations during your clinical postings.

Speed and Volume

Present your history with moderate speed, in a loud and clear voice, taking adequate pause between two lines and sections. Every listener needs some time to understand and imagine about the sufferings about your patient. Even if you have got a good fluency and accent of spoken English, no examiner will be impressed if he is unable to imagine what you are describing about the patient and his disease.

Present as a Speech

Everyone likes to hear a clear and fluent presentation of case history from any student. This can be learnt only by regular practice. To save the precious time, history is mostly noted by students in abbreviated form. But during presentation, it will be better to read it in form of the standard speech. For example:

How to write a case history?

Name: Raju s/o Sunderlal Chhatre

Age/Sex: 35 years/Male

Residence: Village Betma, district Indore

Religion: Marathi, Hindu

Occupation: Laborer in plastic factory

Socioeconomic status (SES): Low

DOA: 25-04-2019

How to read the same case history?

My patient Raju Chhatre, son of Sunderlal Chhatre, is a 35-year-old male. He is a resident of village Betma, district Indore. He belongs to Marathi caste and Hindu religion, is a laborer in plastic factory by occupation, and is from a low socioeconomic class family. He was admitted here on 25th April 2019 with chief complaints of.....

This skill can be achieved and improved only by practice. Try to present as many cases as possible. You can even rehearse to improve your fluency and pronunciation in front of your friends. This will improve your confidence and quality of your presentation.

Eye Contact

Make proper eye contact with the person to whom you are presenting your case. This will make you look impressive and confident during your presentation. Keep it in mind while replying to his questions also.

Avoid Abbreviations

Avoid using nonstandard abbreviations while presenting your case history. This may annoy and irritate your teacher or examiner. For example, it may not be liked by many if you present some patient's past history as *there is no history of TB, DM, HT, or any other significant disease in past*.

Selection of Information

Your patient may give you all types of information about his disease, past, and lifestyle. Try to select only the relevant and significant information for your presentation. Listen everything calmly, but exclude it if you feel that it is insignificant in context of his disease. For example, a female with a lump in her breast may tell you in great details about her constipation, but you present about it up to certain extent including only the relevant information. This skill of inclusion and exclusion of information will get better with improvement of your knowledge of various diseases. At the same time, whenever you are having any doubt about the significance of any information, prefer to include it in your presentation.

Question Bank

Try to present and discuss about various types of patients to as many persons as possible like to your teachers, PG residents, interns, etc. This discussion will increase your knowledge about the common questions related to various types of diseases. This will be of great help to you during your practical examinations. Similarly, you should also discuss and share your experience about different cases with your colleagues.

CHAPTER 18

An Illustrated Case History

The most important thing in communication is hearing what isn't said.
—*Peter Drucker*

On 5th June 2019, a female patient was admitted in the surgical ward with a complaint of swelling in her neck. Next day, an undergraduate medical student was asked to take her history for presentation. Following is a verbatim presentation of conversation between the student and the patient.

All names, which have been mentioned in this chapter, are fictitious. Any resemblance with any living or dead person is purely coincidental.

Student: *Namskaar. Aapka naam kya hai?* (Hello. What is your name?)
Patient: *Savitri.* (Savitri)

Student: *Savitri ji, mera naam Ajeet Jain hai. Mujhe bade saheb ne aapse aapki beemari ke bare me kuchh puchhne ke liye bheja hai, jo mai baad me unhe bataane wala hu. Kya abhi aapse baat kar sakta hu?* (Savitri ji, my name is Ajeet Jain. Our senior doctor has asked me to have a talk with you about your disease. I will discuss with him about it later. Can we talk right now?)
Patient: *Jee, sir.* (Yes sir)

Student: *Aapko kya takleef hui hai?* (What is your complaint?)
Patient: *Yeh gathan ho gayi hai.* (I have got a swelling here.)
(She pointed toward a swelling at the left side of her neck.)

Student: *Aapke saath yeh kaun hai?* (Who is she with you?)
Patient: *Jee yeh meri badi behan hai.* (She is my elder sister.)
(Her sister greeted the student and he responded in the same way.)

Student: *Theek. Aapka pura naam kya hai?* (OK. What is your full name?)
Patient: *Savitri Koge.* (Savirti Koge)

Section 4: Student–Patient Interaction

Student: *Aapke pitaji ka naam?* (What is your father's name?)
Patient: *Ramsingh Koge.* (Ramsingh Koge)

Student: *Aapki umra kitni hai?* (How old are you?)
Patient: *19 saal.* (19 years)

Student: *Aap kaha rehti hai?* (Where do you live?)
Patient: *Balwada gaanv me.* (I am from Balwada village.)

Student: *Yeh kis jile me hai?* (It is in which district?)
Patient: *Khargone jile me.* (In Khargone district.)

Student: *Aap kis jaati ki hai?* (You belong to which caste?)
Patient: *Balai jaati ki.* (Balai caste.)

Student: *Aap kya kaam karti hai?* (What do you do?)
Patient: *Jee, majdoori karti hu.* (I am a laborer.)

Student: *Kaha par majdoori karti hai?* (Where do you work?)
Patient: *Chune ki khadaan me.* (In a limestone mine.)

Student: *Aapko kitni majdoori milti hai?* (What are your wages?)
Patient: *Roj ke 150 ₹ milte hai.* (₹ 150 per day.)

Student: *Aap kaha tak padhi hai?* (Till what standard have you studied?)
Patient: *Paanchvi tak.* (I have studied up to 5th standard.)

Student: *Aap yaha kab bharti hui thi?* (When were you admitted in this hospital?)
Patient: *Kal bharti hui thi, sir.* (I was admitted here yesterday.)

Student: *Aapko yeh gathan ki takleef kab se hai?* (Since how long are you having this swelling?)
Patient: *Jee, 2 mahine se.* (For 2 months.)

Student: *Iske alawa koi aur takleef?* (Do you have any other complaints?)
Patient: *Jee, sir. Bukhaar bhi aata hai.* (Yes sir. I am suffering from fever also.)

Student: *Kab se aa raha hai?* (Since how long?)
Patient: *Holi ke baad se.* (Since Holi.)

Student: *Matlab 3 mahine se?* (You mean for 3 months?)
Patient: *Jee sir.* (Yes sir)

Student: *Kya us ke pehle aap bilkul theek thi?* (Were you perfectly alright before that?)
Patient: *Jee sir.* (Yes sir)

Student: *Theek. Ab aap shuruat se apni takleef ke baare me bataiye.* (OK. Now please tell me about your complaints right from the beginning.)
Patient: *Jee, sir. Holi par mai apne mama ke ghar rehne Dewas gayi thi. Wahi par bukhar aana shuru hua. Pehle kuchh din laga ki shayad holi khelne se aa raha hoga. Lekin jab theek nahi hua to maine apne gaanv ke doctor ko dikhaya. Jab tak unki dava leti thi, tab tak theek rehta tha. Lekin dava band karne ke baad phir bukhaar aana shuru ho jata hai.*
(Sir, I had visited Dewas at my uncle's home on Holi. There, I started suffering from fever. For first few days, I thought that it was perhaps because of playing Holi. But when it continued, I consulted a doctor in my village. I felt fine as long as I continued his medicines, but when I stopped them the fever recurred.)
(The student allowed her to speak without any interruption. When she stopped speaking, he asked her the next question.)

Student: *Bukhar kaisa aata hai?* (How is your fever?)
Patient: *Shaam ke samay halka bukhar chad jaata hai.* (I get mild fever, especially in the evening.)

Student: *Theek. Ab is gathan ke baare me kuchh bataiye.* (OK. Now please tell me something about this swelling.)
Patient: *Jee, ye do mahine se hai. Pehle chhoti si thi. Phir dheere dheere badti ja rahi hai.* (It is since the last 2 months. First, it was of smaller size but it is now enlarging gradually.)
(She indicated the initial size of her swelling with her thumb and the index finger.)

Student: *Kya aapko is gathaan se koi takleef hoti hai?* (Do you have any other problem with this swelling?)
Patient: *Jee nahi, sir.* (No, sir.)

Student: *Kya aapko isme dard hota hai?* (Do you feel any pain in it?)
Patient: *Jee nahi sir.* (No, sir.)

Student: *Aur koi takleef? Jaise khana khane me ya saans lene me takleef, ya aavaz me koi fark?* (Do you have any other complaints? Like difficulty in swallowing or breathing, or any change in voice?)

Patient: *Jee nahi sir* (No, sir.)

Student: *Kya aapne is gathan ke liye kahi aur ilaaj liya tha?* (Did you consult someone else for this swelling?)
Patient: *Jee sir. Gaon ke doctor ko hi dikhaya tha. Lekin unki dava se is par koi asar nahi pada.* (Yes sir. I had consulted the same doctor in my village but his medicines did not bring any relief.)

Student: *Matlab aapko 3 mahine se sham ke samay halka bukhaar rehta hai. Aur 2 mahine se aapke gale me yah gathaan ho gayi hai, jo dheere dheere badti ja rahi hai. Aapne iske liye apne gaanv ke doctor se dava li thi. Us se bukhar to kam ho jata tha, lekin gathaan me koi fark nahi pada. Theek?* (OK. So you want to say that you are suffering from fever for 3 months which is mild and occurs in evening. Then you developed this swelling in your neck for 2 months which is gradually increasing in size. You consulted for your problems to a doctor in your village. His medicines relieved your fever but this swelling continued to increase. Right?)
Patient: *Jee sir.* (Yes sir.)
(After this, the student noted down the information in section of "history of presenting complaints" on his sheet.)

Student: *Theek. Kya aapko iske alava kabhi koi aur badi beemari hui hai? Jaise TB ki beemari, blood pressure, shakkar ki beemari ya koi aur beemari?* (OK. Now please tell me that did you ever suffer from any other major problem in the past? Like TB, diabetes, hypertension or any other disease?)
Patient: *Jee nahi, sir.* (No sir.)

Student: *Kya kabhi aapka koi operation hua hai?* (Were you ever operated for any problem in the past?)
Patient: *Jee. Appendix ka operation hua tha. Jab mai 9 saal ki thi.* (Yes sir. My appendix was removed when I was 9 years old.)

Student: *Kya aap iske alawa kabhi kisi asptaal me bharti hui thi?* (Apart from this, were you ever hospitalized for any problem?)
Patient: *Jee nahi, sir.* (No sir.)

Student: *Kya aapko iske pehle is jagah par ya shareer me kahi aur aisi gathaan hui hai?* (Did you ever notice any such swelling here or at any other site of your body?)
Patient: *Jee nahi.* (No sir.)

Student: *Theek. Yeh to aapki beemari ke bare me tha. Ab mai aapse aapki roz ki zindagi aur khan-paan ke bare me kuchh puchhna chahunga.*

(OK. So this was all about your disease. Now I would like to ask few questions about your routine life.)
Patient: *Jee sir.* (OK, sir.)

Student: *Aapko neend kaisi aati hai?* (How is your sleep?)
Patient: *Theek aati hai, sir.* (It is fine, sir.)

Student: *Bhukh kaisi lagti hai?* (How is your appetite?)
Patient: *Jee, aajkal bhukh thodi kam ho gayi hai.* (It has decreased now.)

Student: *Kab se?* (Since how long?)
Patient: *Jab se bukhaar aa raha hai.* (Since the time I am suffering from fever.)

Student: *Khaane me aap kya leti hai? Sirf saag-bhaaji khati hai ya maans-machhli bhi khati hai?* (Are you vegetarian or nonvegetarian?)
Patient: *Jee nahi, sir. Sirf saag-sabji hi khaati hu.* (I am a vegetarian.)

Student: *Khaane me mirch-masala kaisa leti hai?* (Do you prefer spicy food or nonspicy food?)
Patient: *Teekha khaana achchha lagta hai.* (I like spicy food.)

Student: *Ghar me namak kaunsa istmaal hota hai?* (Which salt is used in your family?)
Patient: *Packet wala, Tata ka.* (Packet salt of Tata company.)

Student: *Kya kuchh samay se aapke vajan me koi fark aaya hai?* (Is there any change in your weight?)
Patient: *Jee nahi, sir. Utna hi hai.* (No sir.)

Student: *Kya aapko paan-supaari ya kuchh aur khane ki aadat hai?* (Do you have any habit of eating paan, supaari or anything else?)
Patient: *Jee nahi, sir.* (No sir.)

Student: *Aapko tatti ya pishaab me koi takleef?* (Do you have any problem in urination or motion?)
Patient: *Jee nahi.* (No sir.)

Student: *Kya aapki shaadi ho gayi hai?* (Are you married?)
Patient: *Nahi sir.* (No sir.)

Student: *Theek. Kya aapke pariwar me kisi aur ko aisi ya koi aur badi beemari hui hai?* (OK. Has any other member of your family suffered from similar or any other major illness?)
Patient: *Jee. Chaar mahine pehle mere pitaji ko khaansi aur bukhar ki takleef hui thi. Khargone me jaanch karvaai to TB ki beemari ka*

pata chala. Abhi unka ilaaj chal raha hai. (Yes sir. Four months ago, my father had developed cough and fever. He was diagnosed to be suffering from TB in Khargone. Presently, his treatment is going on.)

Student: *Theek. Ab aapke maasik ke bare kuchh puchhna chahunga. Kya aapka mahina theek aa raha hai?* (OK. Now I would like to ask about your menstruation. Is it going on properly?)
Patient: *Jee sir. Theek se aa raha hai. Koi takleef nahi hai.* (Yes sir. It is fine. I do not have any problem with it.)

Student: *Kitni umra se aana shuru hua tha?* (At what age did your menstruation start?)
Patient: *Jab mai 11 saal ki thi.* (When I was 11 years old.)

Student: *Aakhri baar kab aaya tha?* (When did it come for the last time?)
Patient: *Jee, 2 tareekh ko aaya tha.* (On 2nd of this month.)

Student: *Kitne din me aata hai aur kitne din chalta hai?* (In how many days does it occur? And for how many days does it continue?)
Patient: *30 din me aata hai aur 4 din tak rehta hai.* (It occurs in every 30 days and continues for 4 days.)

Student: *Theek. Kya aap abhi kisi takleef ke liye koi dava le rhai hai?* (OK. Are you taking any medicine for any disease at present?)
Patient: *Jee sir. muhanse ke liye ek ayurvedic dava le rahi hu, 6 mahine se. Uska naam to yaad nahi hai* (Yes sir. I am taking an ayurvedic medicine for my pimples for 6 months but I do not remember its name.)

Student: *Koi baat nahi. Kya aapko kabhi kisi dava se koi takleef hui hai? Jaise khujli, shareer par daane ya koi aur takleef?* (OK. No problem. Did you ever suffer from any reaction after taking any medicine, like itching, rashes or any other problem?)
Patient: *Jee nahi, sir.* (No sir.)

After finishing the case history, the student performed a meticulous general, systemic and local examination of the patient. Then he concluded the conversation as:
Student: *Theek Savitri ji. Dhanyavaad. Mai aapki beemari ke baare me bade sahab ko bata dunga. Aap chinta na kare, bilkul theek ho jaayengi.* (OK Savitri ji. Thank you. I will discuss about your problem with our senior doctor. Don't worry, you will be alright soon.)
Patient: *Jee, Dhanyavad sir.* (Thank you, sir.)

Chapter 18: An Illustrated Case History

▌PRESENTATION OF CASE HISTORY

Case history of this patient was presented by the student as following:

"My patient, Savitri Koge d/o Ramsingh Koge, is a 19-year-old female. She is a resident of village Balwada, district Khargone. She belongs to Hindu religion and Balai caste. She is a laborer in a limestone mine by occupation. She is educated up to 5th standard and belongs to low socioeconomic class.

She was admitted here on 5th June 2019 with chief complaints of:
- Fever since 3 months
- Swelling at left side of neck since 2 months

My patient was apparently alright 3 months back, when she developed fever, which was of low grade and occurred in the evening time. She consulted a doctor at her village who prescribed some medicines for it. Her fever was controlled as long as she continued the medicines but recurred when the treatment was stopped. Around 2 months back, she accidently noticed a small swelling of about 1 cm size on the left side of her neck. It was painless and gradually increased in size. She had consulted the same doctor for the swelling, but his medicines did not bring any change in size or progression of the swelling.

Apart from these, there is no history of pain, dysphagia, dyspnea, voice change or any other significant complaint.

There is no history of tuberculosis, diabetes, hypertension or any other significant chronic illness. Her appendectomy was done around 10 years back. Apart from this, there is no history of hospitalization for any other illness. She has not suffered from similar swelling in the past, at same or at any other site of the body.

Her sleep and appetite are adequate. She is vegetarian, prefers spicy food, and consumes iodized salt. There is no history of any change in her weight and she has got no addiction. Her bladder and bowel habits are normal and she is unmarried.

Her father had suffered from cough and fever 4 months back. He was diagnosed as a case of tuberculosis and presently he is receiving treatment for it. Apart from this, there is no history of similar or any other significant disease to any other member of her family.

She had attained her menarche at the age of 11 years. Her last menstrual period had occurred on 2nd June. Her menstruation is regular, occurs in every 30 days, and continues for 4 days. There is no significant problem associated with her menstrual cycles.

She is taking some ayurvedic medicines for her acne for 6 months. She is not allergic to any drug.

On examination, my patient is found to be conscious, cooperative and well oriented to time, place, and person. Her general condition is good. She is thin built and her nutrition is adequate. She is afebrile, her pulse is 76 beats/min, respiratory rate is 16 per min, regular and her blood pressure is 126/80 mm Hg. She has mild pallor; otherwise she has no icterus, cyanosis, clubbing, edema or lymphadenopathy. Her jugular venous pressure is normal.

On her systemic examination, the examination of her central nervous system is found to be normal. Her apex beat is normally located, S1 and S2 sounds are normal and no murmur was heard during auscultation. Air entry is equal in both the lungs and there are no adventitious sounds. Her abdomen is soft, nontender, and there is no distension or organomegaly.

On local examination, a swelling is visible at anterior triangle of left side of her neck. It is ovoid in shape and of approximately 5 cm × 4 cm size. It has got smooth surface and well-defined regular margins. Skin over the swelling is normal. There are no visible pulsations or cough impulse, and it does not move with deglutition.

On palpation, swelling is found to be located in the region of carotid triangle of the left side of her neck, anterior to sternocleidomastoid muscle. Temperature of skin over the swelling is normal and it is nontender. Its surface is smooth and margins are well-defined and regular. Its size is 5 cm in vertical direction, 4 cm in horizontal direction, and 2.5 cm in maximum height. Consistency is uniformly soft and cystic, fluctuation test is positive, and transillumination test is negative. No pulsations or cough impulse is felt during palpation. Swelling is free from overlying skin and is fixed to the deeper structures. Apart for this, no other swelling is felt during palpation of her neck. Swelling is dull on percussion and no abnormal sound is heard on auscultation over the swelling.

(After this presentation, examiner asked the student about the most probable diagnosis. On the basis of symptoms and signs, he was able to make a clinical diagnosis of "cold abscess in neck".)

Section 5

Six Skills of Communication in Clinical Practice

Section Outline

- ❖ Listening Skills
- ❖ Questioning Skills
- ❖ Answering Skills
- ❖ Explanation Skills
- ❖ Persuasion Skills
- ❖ Examination Skills

CHAPTER 19

Listening Skills

If we were supposed to talk more than we listen, we would have two tongues and one ear.
—Mark Twain

Doctor-patient communication is a two-way interactive communication, as both the doctor and the patient play the roles of speaker and listener. During the initial part of conversation, when patient tells his doctor about his complaints, doctor has to play the role of a good listener. Later on, when he explains the patient about the disease and its management plan, he becomes the major speaker.

In several studies, it was found that one of the common complaints of the patients was that their doctor did not listen to them properly. This brings a sense of major dissatisfaction to many patients. As a result, instead of following their doctor's opinion, many of them prefer to take a second opinion from someone else.

But, for most of the times, this complaint is only because of the poor listening skills of the doctor. Every doctor tries to listen to the complaints of his patient calmly and attentively. But, if he is not aware of his listening skills, patient may misinterpret him as careless and disinterested in listening to his problems.

Following are some important suggestions which will help the doctor to look like a good listener to their patients:

- *Sprinter's position:* While listening to the patient, sit in a slightly forward bending position, with your hands resting on the table. This is known as "Sprinter's position" (**Fig. 19.1**). It brings the listener nearer to the speaker, which makes him feel that the person is relaxed and very much interested in listening to his complaints. Similarly, face-to-face orientation is always better for communication than face-to-side position. This position of the doctor encourages the patient to speak openly about his disease.
- *Eye contact:* Maintain a proper eye contact with your patient during listening. If you frequently look at some different places

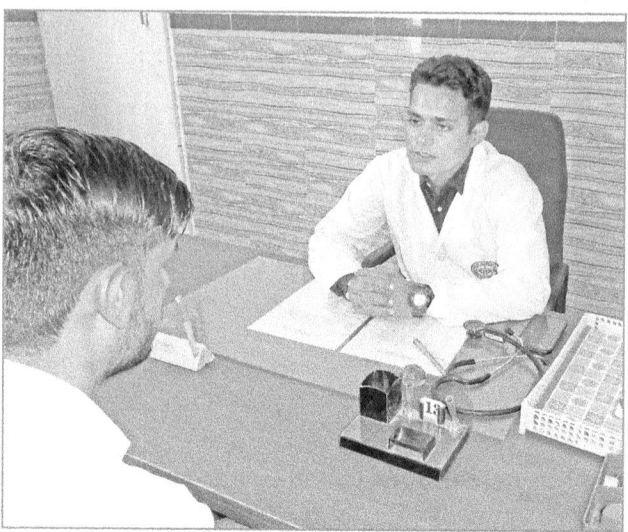

Fig. 19.1: Sprinter's position: Right posture.

(such as ceiling, wall clock, or any other object) for a long time, he may feel that you are not interested and want to finish him as early as possible (**Fig. 19.2**). But at the same time, do not stare continuously at your patient. Some studies suggest that eye contact should be maintained for approximately 70% of time during speaking and 90% of time during listening. Make some intentional breaks during listening, as a constant stare may get some patients uncomfortable, especially of the opposite gender.

- *Head nodding:* Keep nodding you head intermittently. This will encourage your patient to speak out more about his problems.
- *Vocal cues:* Similarly, intermittent vocal cues will also make him feel that you are very much interested in knowing more about his complaints. Vocal cues are various types of humming nonverbal sounds produced by vocal cords during conversation.
- *Facial expressions:* Pay some attention on your facial expressions while listening. Human face can make more than 250 types of different expressions, which are created by various combinations of expressions on forehead, eyebrows, eyes, and lips. During routine communications, these expressions are almost always controlled subconsciously. By paying some attention, doctor can create different types of expressions (such as amazed, thinking,

Chapter 19: Listening Skills

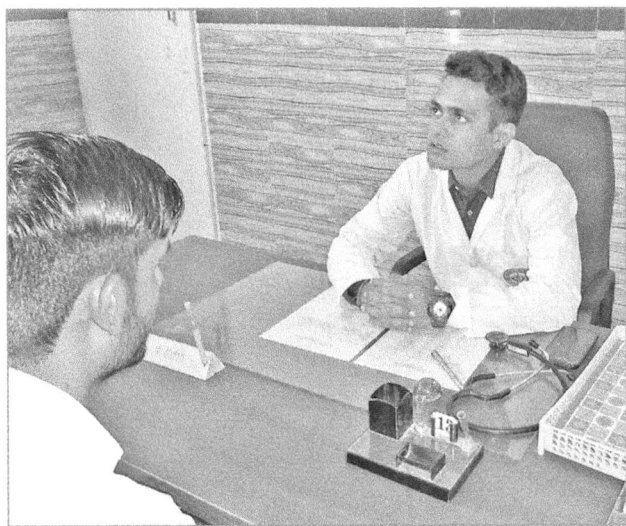

Fig. 19.2: Eye aversion: Poor eye contact during communication.

feeling pity, etc.), according to the type of information received from the patient (**Fig. 19.3**). This will give him a feeling that he is being heard by the doctor attentively. In contrast, if a doctor listens to his patient with an expressionless and mask-like face, after sometime, the patient may start having doubt on the attention and interest of the doctor.
- *Avoid distracters:* Avoid any type of distraction during communication with patients. Some common examples are noises from other persons, fan, mobile phones, etc. If possible, communicate with your patient in a quiet and isolated place. Keep your mobile with your assistant or on vibration mode.

While listening to your patients, avoid making distracting movements, such as fidgeting, foot shaking, clicking the pen, revolving the paper weight, etc. These repetitive nonpurposeful movements are known as adapters. They mostly occur subconsciously and may make your patient feel that you are not interested in listening to his complaints (**Fig. 19.4**).

These all are the examples of external distracters. The more important is to eliminate the internal distracter, which can be simply explained as *thinking of something else* while listening to the patient.

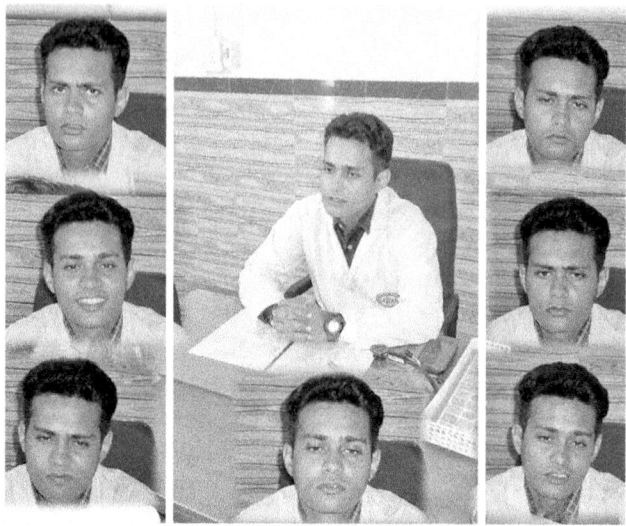

Fig. 19.3: Various types of facial expressions.

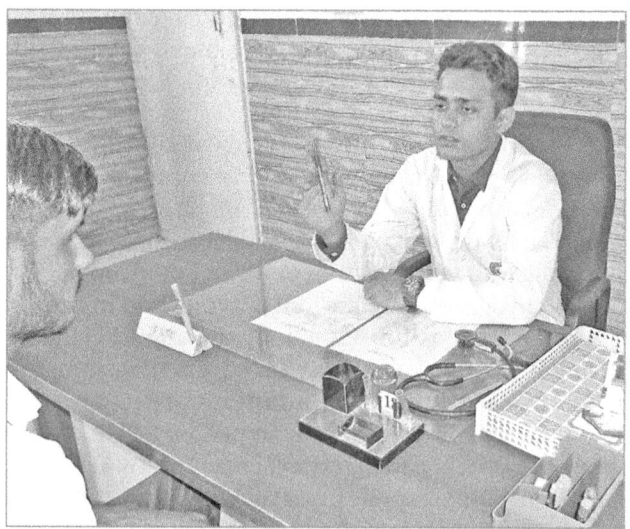

Fig. 19.4: Adapter: Fidgeting with pen.

> A young female patient visited to a physician with complaint of weakness and abdominal pain since last few months. She had already taken several remedies for it. While she was telling him about the course of her illness, she noticed that doctor was not making proper eye contact with her. For most of the time, he was looking at *something* on the roof or the wall behind her. He was sitting leaning backward in his chair and was continuously fidgeting with his pen. Also, he had a single blank expression on his face. Although he was listening to her very attentively, the patient was not sure about his attention and interest. He advised her some investigations and treatment, but she preferred to consult some other doctor for her ailments.

- *Let the patient speak first:* Avoid interrupting the patient while he is telling you about his complaints. A study had revealed that on an average, a patient's speech is interrupted by the doctor within 18 seconds. Same study also showed that an average patient, if allowed to say what he has to say uninterrupted, finishes his story in 90 seconds.

  There are several reasons for why a doctor interrupts his patient from speaking:
  - Shortage of time due to large number of patients.
  - Some patients are talkative by nature. Doctor has to interrupt them whenever their speech gets diverted toward the lengthy and irrelevant information.
  - In some cases, doctor already knows that what patient wants to say. This happens when an experienced doctor meets some patient with a very common disease.

- *Avoid writing simultaneously: You cannot truly listen to anyone and do anything else at the same time*—M Scott Peck.

  The act of writing is essential, but it itself acts as a major distracter during communication with patients. During writing, the doctor is unable to make proper positive signs of communication (such as head nodding, eye contact, facial expressions, etc.) with the patient. So, if possible, first listen attentively to all complaints of your patient and write them down only after presenting him a summary of the information received.

- *Present back a summary:* After listening to his all problems, present the patient a summary of all the information which you have received. In his short speech, patient discloses about multiple information related to his disease, ranging from the most significant to the least significant. Now, after listening them properly, the doctor should rephrase and present the major information back to the patient. For example, after listening to all the complaints of a patient, his doctor presented him a summary like:

So Mr Sharma...You want to say that you have got pain in your right leg since 1 month, which starts after standing for a long time and gets relieved after lying down on bed. And now, you have noticed some swelling in the same leg since last 4 days. Right?

This small act of presenting the summary has got several advantages:
- Patient will reconfirm the information which has been perceived by the doctor.
- He will get an opportunity to clarify or modify any information.
- Most importantly, he will definitely feel that he was well attended and heard by the doctor.

CHAPTER 20

Questioning Skills

Judge a man by his questions rather than his answers
— Voltair

Provisional diagnosis, which is made by the doctor on basis of signs and symptoms of the patient, is greatly influenced by the information provided by the patient about his disease. Accurate information will lead to a correct diagnosis and treatment. In contrast, some wrong or incomplete information may mislead and confuse the doctor.

The amount and reliability of the information provided by the patient mainly depends upon how he has been asked. In other words, the quality of answers given by any patient largely depends upon the quality of questions asked by his doctor. So, it is essential for the doctor to understand the importance of acquiring good questioning skills during communication with his patients.

IMPORTANCE OF QUESTIONING IN COMMUNICATION

During any conversation, the act of asking questions helps a person in following ways:

- Every question is asked to get some answer. They are meant to obtain some information from the other person.
- The person who asks the questions also gains a power to control the conversation. He can guide the whole conversation by changing the type and contents of his questions.
- Questions also show the interest of any person in communication with the other person. The quality of questions shows the curiosity and caring attitude of the person.

■ SELECTION OF RELEVANT QUESTIONS

Questioning is the most primitive skill of communication which is learnt by every doctor right from the beginning of his student life. In fact, this is the only skill which is learnt by him during his study period, because a medical student is not expected to answer or explain anything to his patients. Student gets a standard format of case history which includes a series of different types of questions. Regardless of the disease, he is expected to ask all questions to all patients (comprehensive history taking). Gradually, he learns to select and focus more upon some important questions, according to the type of the disease of his patient (iterative hypothesis testing). For example, a medical student will ask all questions of the standard format to a female patient with a lump in her breast. But, a practicing surgeon will not focus much upon the information which will not be much helpful to him in making her diagnosis or planning her management (e.g., about her occupation, religion, etc.). This art of selection of relevant questions is gradually learnt by the medical student with increasing knowledge about different types of diseases.

Practically, it is very difficult for a practicing doctor to ask all questions to all types of patients because of the following reasons:
- The act of asking everything to everyone will prolong the total duration of communication with a single patient. That will obviously extend the waiting time of the other patients.
- The standard format of history is well-known to the doctors, but not to the patients. Patient may not be able to understand the logic of some questions. For example, a young female with a sebaceous cyst on her forearm may feel perplexed if the doctor asks about her religion, bowel habits, marital status, etc., during very first consultation.
- Sometimes, these questions may divert the attention of doctor and patient in some different direction. For example, a middle-aged female patient presented to an ophthalmologist with complaints of blurring of vision. When he asked about her bowel habits, she started describing about her constipation in great detail. Here, this question was relatively unnecessary as the information of bowel habits is very less likely to play any role in diagnosis and management of blurred vision.

Hence, the selection of questions depends upon the significance of information obtained through them, which varies from disease to disease. In his brief conversation with the patient, doctor is expected to obtain all the relevant information through his questionnaire. This skill of selection of relevant questions increases with time and practical experience of the doctor.

AN IDEAL QUESTION

An *ideal question* from a doctor to his patient should have the following qualities:
- Should be clearly understood by the patient
- Should encourage him to give the maximum possible information
- Should allow him to reply in his own way
- Should not force him to give a highly accurate reply only
- Should not suggest or lead him to give a particular answer

WHY ARE YOU ASKING?

It is essential for a doctor to realize his intention behind asking different types of questions to his patients. The major reason for taking history of any patient is obviously to make a provisional diagnosis of his disease. But, all questions are not intended only for making a diagnosis of the disease. On the basis of their intent, the questions, the standard format of medical history can be divided in following categories:
- Majority of questions help the doctor in making a provisional diagnosis of patient's disease. For example:
  - Upper abdominal pain → Aggravated by: food → Probability of: Gastric ulcer
  - Upper abdominal pain → Relieved by: food → Probability of: Duodenal ulcer
  - Dry gangrene of lower limb → Addiction: Chronic smoking → Probability of: Buerger's disease
  - Pain and swelling of lower limbs → Occupation: Prolonged standing → Probability of: Varicose veins
- Some questions are asked to assess the magnitude and severity of the disease. For example, if the patient is suffering from some painful condition, the major reason behind asking him about his *sleep* is to assess the severity of his pain. Any disease with severe pain will definitely disturb the sleep of the patient. Similarly, a positive history of significant *weight loss* by a patient of suspected malignancy indicates the severity of the tumor.

- Some questions are helpful mainly in planning the management of some conditions. For example, it is important to ask about *diabetes* and *hypertension* to any patient who may need any kind of surgery. Because, a hypertensive patient may be unfit for general anesthesia for some major surgery. Similarly, uncontrolled diabetes may lead to various types of post operative complications such as wound infection, delayed healing, etc. So, it is essential to know about the status and control of these two conditions before planning any type of surgery of the patient. Similarly, the information about the medicines being taken by the patient (*drug history*) and about allergy to any substance (*allergy history*) also help the doctor more in planning the management of his present disease.
- Some questions are practically of not much use in making diagnosis or planning the management of patient's disease. They are mostly asked by medical students during comprehensive history taking, mainly because they are a part of standard format of history taking. For example, asking about religion, residence, sleep, appetite, etc., to a patient with inguinal hernia.

INTERNAL FEELINGS OF THE PATIENT

Different questions bring different types of feelings to different patients. Some questions may be easy and straightforward for them, while some others may be quite difficult and unexpected for some patients. A doctor should be able to anticipate the feelings of any patient when he asks him some question. This will help in framing his questions accordingly; difficult questions are obviously more difficult to ask also.

> A young male presented to a surgical OPD with a swelling at his shoulder region. A female student was asked to take and present his case history. During conversation, he behaved properly as long as she asked about his swelling. But when she asked some questions, such as his food habits, addiction, marital status, etc., he started taking her very casually and asked the similar questions about her personal life. This attitude made the student quite uncomfortable to continue the conversation. This happened because he had visited there for treatment of his swelling and so, he had never expected that a young female doctor will ask him such personal questions.

Chapter 20: Questioning Skills

> A 30-year-old female was admitted with a painless lump in her breast. She was quite comfortable with the consultant in OPD, who had asked her only few specific questions. Soon after her admission, a student took her detailed history in the ward. She became quite uncomfortable when he asked her about her appetite, addiction, bladder and bowel habits, etc., as she was unable to correlate the importance of these questions with her actual problem of breast lump.

Depending upon the significance of questions and preparedness of any patient, the questions of standard format can be broadly divided in three categories. This can be better understood by imagining the example of a female patient who has presented with a painless, slowly growing swelling in front of her neck (which is strongly suspected to be arising from her thyroid gland).

- *Type 1 questions: Relevant for doctor and expected for patient*
  These are simple and straightforward questions. While visiting to the doctor, every patient is usually prepared to answer them. Most of the patients give a confident and straightforward reply to many of these questions. Also, these questions provide some significant information to the doctor for making the diagnosis of the disease. For example, in this case—duration of swelling, progression of swelling, complaint of pain, dysphagia, dyspnea, voice change, etc.
- *Type 2 questions: Relevant for doctor, but unexpected for patient*
  These questions also provide some significant information to the doctor. But, they are mostly surprising and unexpected to the patients. This happens mainly because the patient cannot correlate them with his presenting complaints. He may or may not be able to give a confident and accurate answer to many of such questions. Good questioning skills of doctor will definitely help the patient to give out the best possible answers to such questions. For example, in this case—use of iodized salt, appetite, sleep, weight change, menstrual irregularities, etc. Every doctor knows the importance of these questions in relation to thyroid dysfunctions. But, patient may not be able to correlate their significance in relation to a painless swelling in her neck.
- *Type 3 questions: Irrelevant for doctor and unexpected for patient*
  Although these questions are the part of standard format of medical history, but still the information provided by these

questions is not of much help in making the diagnosis of the disease. Experienced doctors do not usually ask these questions during first conversation with the patients. They are usually asked mainly for the purpose of completing the history sheet of the patient, usually after hospitalization. For example, in this case—religion, vegetarian or non vegetarian, bladder habits, etc.

A medical student asks all three types of questions to all of his patients (comprehensive history taking). But, a practicing physician focuses more upon first two types of questions (iterative hypothesis testing).

TYPES OF QUESTIONS

There are several types of questions which we ask each other during our routine conversation. It is important to ask every question in a proper way, otherwise it may affect the quantity and reliability of the received answer. There are several ways in which the questions can be classified in various types. But, we will focus more upon the following types of questions:
- Open-ended questions
- Closed questions
- Leading questions

- *Open-ended questions:* These are unstructured questions which do not suggest any answer to the patient. He has to reply them in his own words and sentences.
  For example–
  - When does your pain start?
  - How does your pain aggravate?
  - What was the color of vomitus?

  The questions which start with *what, why, where, when, how,* etc. belong to the category of open-ended questions.

- *Closed questions:* In contrast to the open-ended questions, these questions include the answer inside them. Patient has to only give a positive (yes) or negative (no) reply to such questions.
  For example–
  - Does your pain start in evening time?
  - Does your pain aggravate after taking food?
  - Was the vomitus green colored?

  In general, the question which start with *do, does, is, are, was, were, has, have, shall, should, will, would, can, could,* etc., belong to this category.

They expect only a specific answer (yes or no) from the patient. They do not allow him to speak in his own word or sentences. Interestingly, addition of some *options* to an open-ended question converts it to a closed question, as it restricts the freedom of answering openly. For example:
- What was the color of vomitus? Yellow, green or brown?
- How does your pain aggravate? After walking, running or climbing stairs?

Such questions are like double-edged sword; beneficial as well as harmful. In some cases, when patient is unable to understand the question properly, the options help him to understand it by suggesting the possible answers. But at the same time, they may restrict the patient to select any one option from the given list only.

A good questionnaire includes a balanced combination of open-ended and closed questions. No one can take a medical history by using only open-ended or only closed questions. The selection depends upon the personality and understanding of the patient.

Following points should be remembered while asking the questions from the patients:

- Interrogation should always start with open-ended questions. They give a positive feeling to the patient, as he feels that the doctor is giving him an opportunity to speak openly about his problems.
- The information obtained through an open-ended question is more likely to be reliable and accurate. For example, if the patient says that his pain increases with meals in response to an open-ended question (*How does your pain aggravate?*), then it is quite sure that the food is definitely an aggravating factor for his pain. In contrast, if the doctor obtains the same information by asking a closed question (*Does your pain aggravate after meals?*), then a positive answer from the patient may or may not be equally serious and significant.
- Closed questions should be reserved only for the later part of conversations, especially for the situation where open-ended questions are not effective.
- Too many open-ended questions are not suitable for talkative patients, as they find more opportunities to speak out irrelevant or repetitive information. Their speaking can be restricted by using closed questions appropriately.
- Similarly, silent patient also need closed questions more frequently. They may not speak out the desired and adequate information in response to the open-ended questions only.

- *Leading questions:* These questions lead the mind of the patient to a particular answer. They eventually make them feel that the doctor wants to hear only a particular answer from them. For example:
  - Your pain aggravates after taking meals, doesn't it?
  - You are also suffering from constipation, ain't you?
  - You did not have green vomiting, did you?

  Any patient will feel that the doctor wants him to give only the following answers to these questions:
  - Yes. My pain aggravates after meals.
  - Yes. I am also suffering from constipation.
  - No. I did not have green colored vomiting.

  These questions subconsciously lead the mind of the patient to a specific answer, and so, they are called as the leading questions. Such questions should never be used during communication with the patients.

  Interestingly, while asking some questions during our routine talks, we focus more upon the contents and not the types of questions. The type of question mostly comes out spontaneously and subconsciously. To improve his questioning skills, it is important for any doctor to pay some attention toward the selection of the most appropriate type of question for interrogation of his patients.

SINGLE VERSUS MULTIPLE QUESTIONS

The questionnaire of doctor greatly depends upon the response of his patient to his initial questions. During early phase of conversation, doctor subconsciously assesses the understanding, intelligence, language, and speaking habits of his patients, and then plans his questionnaire accordingly.

Speaking habits vary from person to person, ranging from highly talkative to almost silent. Some patients elaborate almost all the information in response to a single question only. In contrast, some patients give only short and specific answer to every question. Both types of patients are almost equally seen in clinical practice. Following example illustrates the communication of a doctor with two different types of patients:

Patient 1:

Dr – "What is your problem?"
Pt 1 – *"I am having pain in my left leg for last 1 month. It starts after walking for some distance and increases as I continue to walk. Sometimes, it becomes so severe that I have to take some rest. Also, I*

am noticing some swelling in this leg since a week. I had consulted my family physician for it. He had prescribed me some medicines, but I was not relieved. So, now he has asked me to consult you for this problem."

Patient 2:

Dr – "What is your problem?"
Pt 2 – *"Pain in my left leg."*

Dr – "Since how long?"
Pt 2 – *"Since 1 month."*

Dr – "OK. Tell me something more about your pain. Is it intermittent or continuous?"
Pt 2 – *"Intermittent."*

Dr – "How does it start?"
Pt 2 – *"Whenever I walk."*

In first case, doctor calmly listens to the information given by the patient. He then asks the remaining information in form of various questions. In contrast, in second case, he will have to ask multiple questions to extract the desired information from the patient.

The quality of information provided by the patient is also variable. Some patients are highly talkative. They enjoy explaining their problem in great details. Most of the information given by them are irrelevant and time consuming. Doctor has to frequently interrupt their speech by introducing some relevant questions. For example:

Dr – "What is your problem?"
Pt 3 – *"Well. Around a month ago, I had visited to my cousin brother, who lives about 100 km away from my place. One evening, I was having a walk with his son. We walked for about 30–35 minutes. Then, I started feeling some pain in my left leg. Firstly, I thought that it must be because of the cloudy weather. So, I asked my wife to massage it with mustard oil, which was quite relieving for me. But next day, I felt the same problem after walking in the market....."*

In short, different patients respond differently to the same question of the doctor. The questionnaire of doctor should be flexible and variable, depending upon the personality and response of the patient.

▌EXTENT OF ENQUIRY

It is important for the doctor to assess the optimum extent of any enquiry while taking history of his patients. The information should be asked up to different extents, depending upon the presenting complaints and suspected diagnosis of the patient. For example, it is important to ask about the *dietary history* of any patient. But, the extent of questioning depends upon the complaints and suspected diagnosis, such as:

- If constipation is the major problem, it will be important to know about the relative amount of fiber diet in his meals. For example: is he vegetarian or nonvegetarian? If nonvegetarian, how frequently does he take nonvegetarian diet? What is the relative amount of nonvegetarian diet in his meals? etc.
- If some parasitic disease, such as cysticercosis is suspected (caused by *Taenia solium*, which is transmitted by improperly cooked pork), the enquiry should be shifted on the type of nonvegetarian food consumed by the patient. Such as: *What do you consume in nonvegetarian food? Have you recently consumed improperly cooked nonvegetarian food at some unknown place?* etc.
- For hypertension and cardiac disease, it will be logical to enquire about the amount of various elements such as fat, carbohydrate, salt, etc., in diet of the patient.
- In cases of suspected thyroid disorder, focus should be made on the type of salt (iodized or noniodized) consumed by the patient.

The questions, which are relevant and informative in one type of patients, may be irrelevant and time-consuming for the other patients. Such as: many other skills, this art of deciding the extent of enquiry improves with the experience of the student and doctor.

HOW TO IMPROVE YOUR QUESTIONING SKILLS?

During communication with his patients, a doctor can improve his questioning skills by taking care of following points:

- Question should be clearly understood by the patient. It should not contain any word which can be missed or misinterpreted by any lay person (e.g., English words, medical words, etc.).
- It should be asked with proper speed, tone, and volume. Speed should be moderate, as any new and unexpected question becomes even more difficult if someone asks it rapidly. Similarly, volume should be moderate, as patient may not like to draw any attention of surrounding persons. If the conversation is going on at some open space, the volume should be further lowered down while asking some personal questions such as addiction, menstrual history, etc.

- Ask only one question at a time. Patient may find it difficult to face multiple questions together. Similarly, it may be difficult for him if any question is followed by multiple options. Such as—

    "Have you suffered from any disease like TB, diabetes, hypertension, asthma, epilepsy, jaundice or anything like that in past?"

- If any patient is unable to understand some question, keep its alternative form ready for him. Some patients may not understand some questions clearly. So, the doctor should instantly rephrase them in some different form. For example:

    Dr – Is there any recent change in your weight?
    Pt – Well....I think....

    Dr – OK. Is there any change in fitting of your clothes in last few weeks or months?
    Pt – Yes sir. I am feeling it difficult to hook my pants nowadays.

- Do not expect an instant answer of every question from your patient. Give him some time to think about it. The average response latency (time span between the stimulus and the reaction) during conversations is approximately 0.5 seconds.
- Similarly, do not ask your next question immediately after the answer of the patient. Take a small break before asking another question, especially if he has given a long answer to your previous question.
- While patient is answering your question, keep encouraging him by positive body language, such as head nodding, eye contact, vocal cue, etc. This will send him a message that he is giving you the appropriate and desired information. In contrast, a blunt expression of the doctor may not encourage him to speak more about his sufferings.
- Before asking another question, try to make some comment on the answer given by the patient to your previous question. Sometimes, even rephrasing the answer of patient makes conversation more interesting and effective. For example:

    Dr – "Do you have any addiction?"
    Pt – "No, sir. I have quitted smoking for last 4 years."

    Dr – "That's very good. Now tell me that for how many years did you smoke before that?"
    Pt – "I smoked for about 20 years, almost 3–4 packets of cigarette every day."

Dr – *"3–4 packets?!" (surprised)*
Pt- "Yes, sir. Then I lost my best friend 4 years ago. He died of lung cancer due to smoking."

Dr- "Oh. That's so unfortunate. But it's good that you've quitted smoking. Did you ever have any other addiction?"
Pt- *"No, sir."*

In other words, instead of making a "question-answer-question-answer" type of plane communication, try to converse on the line of "question-answer-comment-question-answer-comment".

- A good questionnaire includes proper combination of open-ended and closed questions. Start your conversation with open-ended questions. Use closed questions later, only when they are absolutely required.
- Avoid leading questions, as they may forcefully lead patient's answer to a particular direction.
- If patient is unable to give an accurate reply to some question, immediately give him some liberty to give an approximate answer. For example—age of patient, duration of some complaint, time of any significant event in past, etc.

CHAPTER 21

Answering Skills

Wise men speak because they have something to say; Fools because they have to say something
—*Plato*

Communication between a doctor and his patient is a two-way interactive type of communication, where both of them play the role of speaker as well as the listener. First, the doctor listens to the complaints of his patient. Then, he asks him some specific questions. Finally, after examining the patient, he explains him about the provisional diagnosis, required investigations, management, etc. Along with this, during his conversation with the patient, he is also expected to give satisfactory answers of some questions from patient or his relatives. These questions may be of different types, ranging from common to unexpected, from easy to difficult, and from logical to irrational and annoying.

Following are some of the commonly asked questions by patients or their relatives:
- Why has it happened to me? (*Aisa kyo ho gaya hai?*)
- Will I get relieved of my problem? (*Theek to ho jayega na?*)
- Can it happen again? (*Dubara to nahi hoga na?*)
- For how many days will I have to stay in hospital? (*Kitne din bharti rehna hoga?*)
- How much will be the expenditure? (*Kitna kharcha ho jayega?*)

A good doctor should try to develop good answering skills for these common questions. Many of these questions may be difficult, surprising, or annoying for the beginners. But, with increasing experience, the doctor learns to find the most satisfactory answers of such questions.

A reasonable answer to such questions impresses the patient in several ways. He feels that his doctor is quite caring and concerned for his health and well-being. Also, through these answers, he also perceives the knowledge and confidence of his doctor. In contrast, a vague and nonspecific answer may give him a negative feeling for the doctor. He may think that the doctor is either neglecting him or is not very confident regarding his management.

Following are some of the precautions which should be remembered while answering common questions of patients:

1. How to respond to a question?

   Every answer is obviously preceded by some question. The reliability of the answer increases if the person feels that his question was heard properly. So, show proper listening skills (like eye contact, head nodding, vocal cues, etc.) when patient is asking any question. For some questions, it is better to take a small pause before starting the answer. Prompt answers are not always impressive. Occasionally, give a complement to the patient for asking some good question. This will also give him a positive impression for your nature and attitude.

2. *Keep it short and simple:* An ideal answer is the one which succeeds in satisfying the query of the patient. It should not be too long or too short and should not contain any word which is incomprehensible for the patient (e.g., Medical word or English word). Do not forget that it is being given to a layperson and not to some doctor or examiner.

3. *Paraverbal and nonverbal elements:* The reliability of any answer increases if it has been delivered with proper tone and body language. The answer should be fluent and straightforward, without any fillers and fumbles. It should be given maintaining proper eye contact with the patient or his relatives. Similarly, proper attention should be given to the other elements like gestures, facial expressions, etc.

4. *Control your nerves:* Whenever a patient visits his doctor, he tries to get clear answers of maximum possible questions. So, even when the doctor is explaining them properly about the disease, some patients keep on asking different types of questions. Some of these questions only prolong the duration of conversation and distract both of them from the basic line. For example:
   - "How will you remove this tumor from my body?"
   - "How many stitches will be needed in this operation?"
   - "My sodium level is normal. What does sodium do in our body?"

   These questions only arise because of the curiosity and apprehension of the patient. Their answers will not be of very much benefit for him. Doctor should try to keep himself calm and cool during such situation. In fact, if he frequently encounters such questions, he should try to frame a simple straightforward one-liner answer for them.

Chapter 21: Answering Skills

5. *Beyond the limits:* In today's era, the spectrum of medical science has reached to the level of various specialties and super specialties. A doctor, who is expert of his own field, may not be the suitable person to comment upon all types of questions of some other field, but this fact is mostly not known to the patients. They think that *all doctors can treat anything and everything.* So, during or after their consultation with a doctor, they may ask something which is beyond his expertise. This may sometimes lead the patient to a state of confusion and to the doctor in a state of trouble. For example:

> An elderly person visited to a famous cardiologist for his cardiac problem. He was accompanied by his son. Both of them got highly impressed by the behavior, knowledge, and communication skills of the doctor. After his consultation was over, the patient requested the doctor to have a look at a small swelling on shoulder of his son. The cardiologist superficially examined it and asked few questions. The young man told him that the swelling was painless and he was applying some home remedy for it. Instead of advising some investigations or referring him to a surgeon, the doctor verbally advised him to continue the same treatment and report him after few days. Unfortunately, it was a malignant tumor which got advanced in next few weeks. It was realized only when the young male consulted a surgeon. Just to hide their own negligence, both father and the son blamed everything to the cardiologist—"It was *him* who had asked us *to not to do anything*".

In such condition, doctor should go only for a superficial history and examination of the problem (mainly for the satisfaction of the patient) and should clearly explain the patient that the disease is beyond his field and so, he should consult someone else for it.

6. *Importance of words:* Sometimes, it is better to put at least some words with any positive or negative answer. This will give a better impression than by replying only through gestures or vocal cues. This can be understood by imagining the following example on yourself only:

> Imagine that you have got some problem with the vision of your right eye and you have consulted multiple ophthalmologists for it. All of them have unanimously advised a common surgery for it, which is having almost 100% success rate. When you had asked this question to them—*Doctor, will I be able to see through this eye after my surgery?*, they responded as:

> Dr 1—nodded his head, without saying any word.
> Dr 2—nodded his head with a vocal cue (*hu*).
> Dr 3—nodded his head and said—"Yes".
> Dr 4—nodded his head and said—"Yes. You will be able to see everything comfortably".
> Now, as the patient, to whom will you prefer to operate upon your eye?

All of these are affirmative answers, but they have been conveyed to the patient in four different ways. In such condition, responding with little or no words may sometimes give an impression of underconfident attitude of the doctor, especially if he is a young one. In contrast, proper use of some words will impart an impression of confident and caring attitude. Same rule holds true while conveying some negative answer to the patient.

7. *If you do not know the answer:* No doctor is an encyclopedia of medical science. This is a dynamic field which includes enumerable diseases, investigation modalities, treatment lines, etc. So, it is not uncommon for the doctor to come across something which is not very well-known to him. He may need some time to update his knowledge about it. It is true that he should be honest to his patient and should not try anything without proper knowledge and updating. But at the same time, he should understand that his open and honest confession (of not knowing about the disease) may not always give a positive impact to the patient and his relative. For example:

> A young man visited to a surgeon with a painless swelling on his temporal region. It was firm, nontender, and freely mobile. Surgeon suspected it to be fibroma or lipoma and advised for fine-needle aspiration cytology (FNAC). After few days, patient returned to his clinic with cytological report of schwannoma, which was an uncommon (but not very rare) diagnosis. The young surgeon felt himself in trouble as he had got no practical experience of management of schwannoma. So, he honestly confessed as—"Sorry but I do not know much about this disease. So, I will have to first read about it. Can you please see me again tomorrow?". No surprise that patient never came back to him.

It is true that all the doctors cannot treat all the problems equally. It is essential for them to keep learning and updating themselves.

But such a condition, where one has to respond instantly, should be handled trickily. Confessing openly about the lack of knowledge may sometimes horrify the patient, as he may start having doubts on the capability of the doctor. Instead of it, doctor should borrow some time (for reading, net surfing, consulting his colleagues and seniors, etc.) by giving some other reason—*Well. I would like to have a talk with the pathologist about it. Can you please see me again tomorrow?*

8. *Common questions and answers:* Following are some hypothetical examples of different types of answers given to some common questions from patients. Readers are requested to select the best answer out of each set.

Case 1: On knowing about the diagnosis of carcinoma of urinary bladder, an elderly man asked his doctor:

Why has it happened to me, doctor?

Dr 1—"Well. There can be multiple reasons like exposure to some chemicals like dyes, paints, rubber, petroleum products, textiles, or even cigarette smoke also".

Dr 2—"Because you did not take care of your health properly".

Dr 3—"Please focus on the treatment and stop finding the cause".

Dr 4—"Probably because it was in your destiny. No fault from your side".

Case 2: Before her surgery for a malignant tumor, a female patient asked her doctor:

Can it happen again after surgery?

Dr 1—"According to different studies, the recurrence rate of this tumor is from 8.2 to 11.3%".

Dr 2—"No. If I am operating, it will never recur".

Dr 3—"How can I say that? I am not the God".

Dr 4—"Do not worry. Chances are very less. You will be alright".

Case 3: On being hospitalized for enteric fever, a man asked his doctor:

For how many days will I have to be in the hospital?

Dr 1—"How can I say that right now? May be few days or few weeks".

Dr 2—"Stop bothering about the expenditures. Your health is more important than your money".

Dr 3—(in a fun mood) "Take a leave of at least 1 month from your job. It will be less than that".

Dr 4—"It depends on how your body responds to the treatment. Usually, it needs hospitalization for at least 3-4 days".

To summarize, an ideal answer from the doctor should have the following qualities:
- Should satisfy the query of the patient.
- Should be neither too short nor too long.
- Should not contain the difficult and incomprehensible words (like English words or Medical words).
- Should be delivered with polite tone and confident body language.

CHAPTER 22

Explanation Skills

Diagnosis is not the end, but the beginning of practice.
—*Martin H Fischer*

Out of all skills, this is the most important, essential, and difficult skill during communication with the patients. As per our law, patient has got full right to know about the details of his disease (such as the disease, investigations, management, prognosis, etc.), and it is the responsibility of the physician to explain him about it properly, *even if he does not ask about it.*

Following are several advantages of explaining the patient about his disease and plan of management:

- A well explained patient is less likely to go for a second opinion or internet surfing about his disease.
- The act of explaining also brings an opportunity for the doctor to show his confidence in management of the disease. If the doctor explains in a precise and specific way, patient develops faith in him and his line of management.
- In case of an adverse outcome, prior explanation about the disease and management may save the doctor from some major litigation.

> Parents of a child with inguinal hernia had consulted several surgeons for its treatment. The only information, which was given by all of them, was that the child was having a problem of hernia and he would need a surgery for it. Parents were not satisfied and started seeking for some nonoperative remedy for it. Finally, one surgeon explained them properly about *what is hernia? what can be the complications if it is left untreated? what is done in its surgery?*, etc. This information clarified their concepts about the disease of their baby and they decided to get him operated by that surgeon.

The nature of doctor-patient relationship is gradually changing with time, especially in last few decades. Earlier, patients behaved mostly as passive recipients who obeyed all the instructions and remedies provided by their treating doctor. But now, because of increasing knowledge and awareness, the doctor is expected to acquire a patient-centered approach, which is focused at maximum possible involvement of patient and his relatives in taking any major decisions related to his treatment.

In several studies, it was found that the major reason of dissatisfaction of patient's relatives was not the adverse outcome (such as complications, death, etc.), but was the tendency of the doctor to provide very little or no information about the disease and its treatment.

In routine practice, a physician has to commonly inform the patient and his family members about the followings:
- The nature and course of the disease
- Possible complications of the disease
- Investigation plans
- Treatment plans
- Possible complications of the treatment (e.g., side effect of drugs, complications of surgery or anesthesia, etc.)
- Prognosis

But, it is easier to be said than to be done. Following are some of the common difficulties faced by the doctor while explaining the patient about his disease and its management:
- Disparity in the knowledge (of medical science and terminologies) is the most important barrier to communication in this part. It is easier for a doctor to explain about any disease to his colleagues. But the same job becomes very difficult if it is to be done to a lay person, who is not aware of even basic anatomy and physiology of human body.
- Many a times, it becomes difficult to decide about the optimum extent of information that should be explained to the patient. Only superficial and too little information may not be sufficient in some cases. But at the same time, too deep and detailed information may sometimes lead him to a state of misunderstanding and confusion.

These problems are mainly faced by the doctor during early stage of his clinical practice. Gradually, this task becomes less difficult for him with increasing experience.

Following are some important points which should be remembered while explaining the patient about his disease:
- *Right of confidentiality:* Before explaining about the disease, be careful about the presence of relatives along with the patient. As per the right of confidentiality, the information about the disease

Chapter 22: Explanation Skills

of the patient cannot be shared with anyone else without his or her permission (except for few special conditions). So, the choice of relatives who should be included or excluded in this conversation should be left to the patient only. If patient does not want to share about his disease even with his closest family members, his choice should be fully respected.

> A 35-year-old lady visited to a surgeon along with her husband with a painless lump in her breast. After taking proper history and examination, he prescribed her some investigations. After few days, she visited back to him with all the reports (which were indicating toward the malignancy). But this time, due to some reasons, her husband could not come and so she was accompanied by her mother. After reading all the reports, the young surgeon started explaining her about the disease and its management in presence of her mother. The old lady was hypertensive and so, her daughter never wished her to hear any bad news about her disease. Now, for next few days, the major problem of the lady was shifted from her breast lump to the hypertension of her mother.

Although a doctor knows better about the disease, but still, a patient knows better about his family.

- *Check his knowledge about the disease:* It is quite common for the patients to take multiple consultations and opinions for their diseases. Many a times, before consulting the doctor, patient may have consulted someone else for the same problem. Similarly, internet surfing may be another source of this knowledge. So, before explaining him about his disease, it is better to enquire about his knowledge about it. This will help the doctor in focusing upon the important and missing points, as he can confirm or correct the information already acquired by the patient.

> A young female with multiple gallstones visited to a laparoscopic surgeon. The stones were asymptomatic and were incidentally diagnosed few months ago. When the surgeon asked her about any treatment history, she denied for any previous consultation. Surgeon could not believe it, and so, asked her again. With some hesitation, she accepted that she had taken several home remedies and alternative medicines. Also, she had consulted two more surgeons recently, and both of them had advised for surgical removal of her gallbladder. Since she was not convinced, she was

> seeking for some conservative treatment for her stones. All these information helped the surgeon in designing his explanation, and he focused more on what was not known to the patient. Finally, she was convinced and underwent laparoscopic cholecystectomy after few days.

Nowadays, it has become a common habit of the patients to check everything on internet. No one can stop them from accessing the freely available online material. A huge amount of information is available there, even on the very small and trivial topics. But unfortunately, the authenticity of the available information is not always accurate. Moreover, some patients may get confused by searching the same information from multiple sources. Some others may get frightened by the statistical figures of complications of disease or treatment.

During his consultation, the doctor gets an opportunity to check and if required, correct such knowledge of his patient. Whenever he comes across such condition, he should calmly explain the patient about the real fact, and should advise him to avoid random surfing on sensitive topics in future.

- *Gentle, polite, and confident:* Many a times, the real combat of doctor occurs with some illogical beliefs of patient. Some patients make their own assumptions and logics, which are difficult to be corrected. There can occur a conflict between the logics of medical science and irrational thinking of patients.

> Parents of a 7-month-old child noticed a swelling in his scrotum since few days. They consulted his pediatrician, who referred him to a surgeon. After finishing his examination, the surgeon was about to start his explanation. Before he could speak anything, child's father started describing his own logics. "I knew that this was going to happen. We had told the gynecologist to try for normal labor, but she insisted us for cesarean delivery. I am also not happy with the pediatrician. Last month, he carelessly gave some vaccine in his thigh. See, the swelling is on same side." Finally, he looked at the mother – "I have also told her to burp him properly after every feed. But, she never cares about it." The surgeon was speechless, as he had never heard any of those three reasons as the etiology of pediatric hydrocele.

A doctor should try his best to be gentle and calm in such situations. Some of such logics can be ignored, but some others need a correction. He should politely explain the patient and relatives about the real reasons and facts. His politeness and confidence will certainly help him in clearing their misconceptions. In contrast, heated arguments may sometimes lead to some unpleasant situations.

- *Language:* At any stage of doctor-patient communication, the importance of language should not be ignored. Even if the doctor explains everything to the patient, he will be unable to understand anything if the explanation is full of words which are unknown for him (e.g., Medical terminologies, English words, etc.). Many a times, such words are used subconsciously during conversation. Avoid the use of Medical terms and try to replace them with some well-known and easily understood words. Similarly, the commonly spoken English words should be used only after assessing the intellectual level of the patient.

> An elderly female was operated for carcinoma breast. Modified radical mastectomy was performed and specimen was sent for biopsy. The report revealed it to be a grade 3 ductal carcinoma, but axillary lymph nodes were not involved. The consultant asked the PG student to explain about the further management to her family. He called her son, who was a carpenter and educated up to 8th standard. He explained him as – *"Aaapki mataji ki biopsy report me cancer aaya hai, jo bahut high grade ka hai. Lekin unki kismat achchhi hai ki vo abhi tak unki lymph nodes tak nahi pahucha hai. Abhi kuchh dino ke baad hum unki chemotherapy shuru karenge."* ("Biopsy report of your mother has revealed that she was having a cancer of very high grade. But she is lucky because it has still not reached to her lymph nodes. Now, we will start her chemotherapy after few days"). No doubt that her son was unable to understand anything about the disease or management plan of her mother.

The understanding and intellectual level of any patient can be perceived during initial few minutes of the conversation. Many a times, this does not match with the appearance of the patient. So, the doctor should silently assess some factors of his personality (such as perception power, knowledge of English language) during the initial part of the communication. This will help him in tailoring his explanation speech accordingly.

- *Paraverbal elements:* Various elements of paraverbal communication (such as speed, volume, tone, etc.) play an important role in overall outcome of doctor-patient communication. Explanation should be done with moderate volume and speed, as the information is totally new for the patient and so, he will need some time to receive and interpret it.

  The tone of explanation should be of adult-to-adult type, and not like parent-to-child type. It is obviously true that the doctor has got much more knowledge of the disease of his patient. But still, sometimes patients get offended if they are being explained like small kids, especially by some young doctor.

  Instead of making a stereotyped nonstop speech, doctor should take some deliberate *pauses* after few sentences. A good speaker takes short pause after some important statement (as practiced by some famous politicians). This gives few moments to the listeners to think about and feel the importance of the statement. Similarly, the gravity of some statement can be increased by putting *stress* on the important words in it. For example, the impact of this statement—"You will not be able to walk for at least 4 days after the surgery" will be certainly increased if the doctor puts some stress on just two words—"not" and "four".

- *Nonverbal elements:* Several elements of body language play a major role in improving the explanation skills, most important are gestures and eye contact.

  Communicate with your patients in an open posture. Both hands should be kept free. Some common errors are: Keeping one or both hands in pocket (of trouser or apron), arms folded in front of the chest, hands crossed behind or in front of the groin region, etc. **(Figs. 22.1 to 22.3)**. Some of these wrong positions are known as closed or defensive postures and are not considered good during communication.

  The major advantage of acquiring an open posture is that the hands are free for making *conversational gestures*. These gestures are the random movements of one or both hands which are made subconsciously by the person during his speech **(Fig. 22.4)**. Since they are made only when the person speaks, they are named as the conversational gesture. Properly made conversational gestures make a great emphasis on the conveyed information or advice. (You can imagine a person explaining you something with both hands in his pocket, and another person explaining the same thing with proper conversational gestures). The practice and quality

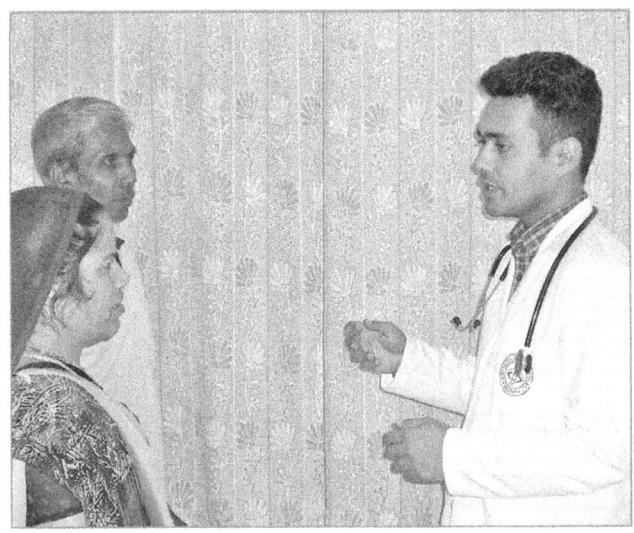

Fig. 22.1: Open posture.

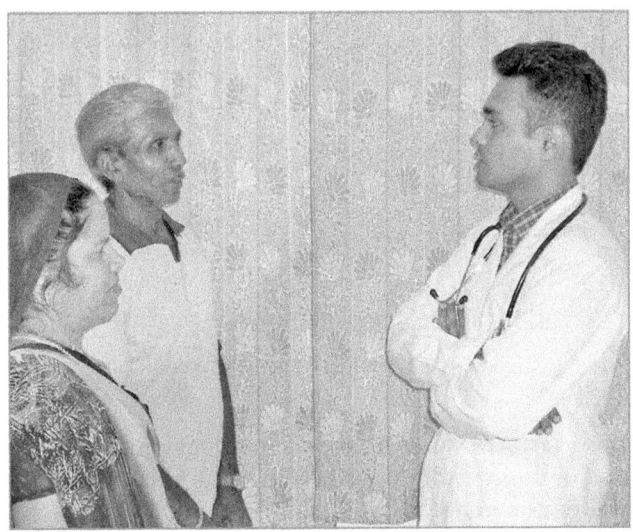

Fig. 22.2: Closed posture.

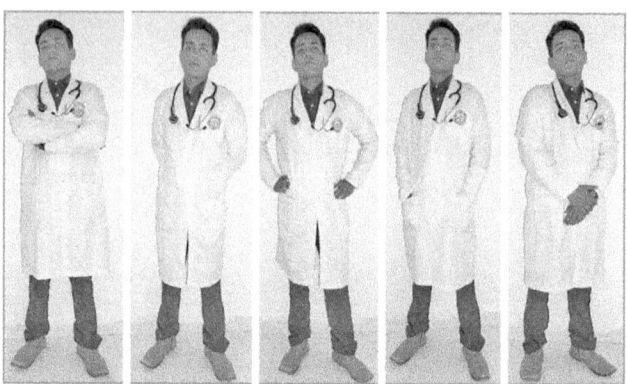

Fig. 22.3: Various types of wrong postures in standing position.

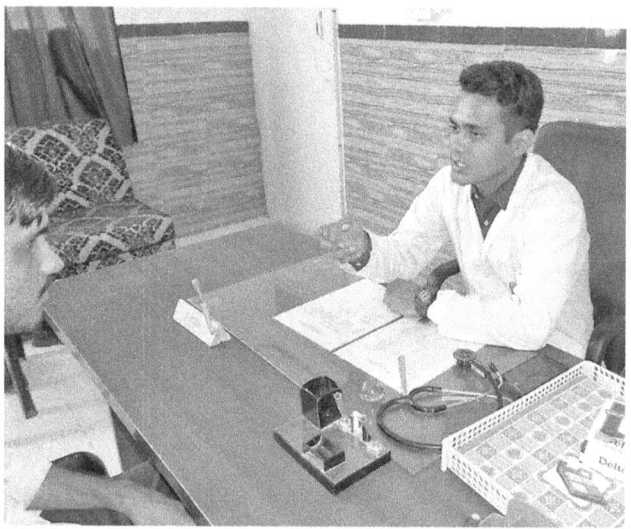

Fig. 22.4: Conversation gestures.

of these gestures varies from person to person. But, they can be started or improved by anyone with some attention and practice of his body language.

While explaining him about his disease, it is important for the doctor to maintain a proper eye contact with his patient **(Fig. 22.1)**. Some studies state that the speaker should maintain an eye contact with his listener for about 70% of time of his speech. As with the other elements, this parameter also varies from person to person. Someone who speaks with proper eye contact looks more confident and reliable to the listener. In contrast, if little or no eye contact is made (known as eye aversion), the listener starts having doubt on the confidence of the speaker.

In this regard, it should be remembered that if the patient is accompanied by one or more relatives, doctor should not focus his eyes on the patient only. Many a times, others start feeling neglected during conversation. Instead of it, he should intermittently look at the accompanying persons, according to their relative importance in management of patient's disease.

> A young lady visited to a female gynecologist for some menstrual problem. She was accompanied by her husband. While the couple was sitting in front of the doctor, she focused all her communication with the patient only. Even while explaining her about the problem and its management, she hardly looked at her husband. Though the patient was very much satisfied, still her husband insisted her to take another opinion, only because he was feeling totally neglected during consultation.

Though the facial expressions play more important role during listening, their significance cannot be ignored during speaking also. The speech of doctor's explanation may contain various types of positive and negative information. It will be better if they are spoken with appropriate expressions on his face.

- *Images speak better than words:* As mentioned earlier, patient's lack of knowledge of medical science is an important barrier in his communication with the doctor. In many cases, when the doctor explains about the disease, patient has to imagine about the pathological changes in relation to the particular organ or body part. This is not an easy task for a lay person, and so, he may not be able to understand the conveyed information properly.

This barrier can be effectively overcome by simultaneous use of various display materials such as charts, dummies, videos, power points presentations, etc. Even if nothing is available, doctor can simply make instant diagrams of the involved organ system. This method will also help in explaining about the plan of management, especially in surgical cases. Also, it will improve the understanding of the patient, as he will not have to make imaginations out of the spoken words.

> A young male patient visited an urologist with his ultrasonography report which was revealing an impacted stone in his ureter with mild hydronephrosis of his right kidney. He had already consulted few more doctors, but was not satisfied with them. In his clinic, urologist explained him about the problem, possible complications, and the management with the help of a dummy (of urogenital system) and a small animation (on ureteroscopic removal of stone). This made everything clear to the patient and he readily accepted the advised treatment.
>
> Same evening, the urologist was called for his opinion for a hospitalized patient with almost same problem and diagnosis. There, he explained all these things to patient and his relatives by drawing a rough diagram on a paper sheet. The teaching method was different, but outcome was the same.

- *Use of analogies:* In some situations, doctor is able to correlate the medical information with some simple example from the routine life of the patient. If used appropriately, this method can improve the understanding of patient in a very simple but effective way.

> A rural patient presented to a surgeon with a tender swelling in his submandibular region. Clinical examination and investigations indicted toward a diagnosis of submandibular lymphadenitis, with a very small amount of pus among the inflamed lymph nodes. Surgeon explained him about the disease and the line of management. Since there was no significant suppuration, surgeon preferred to treat it conservatively and explained him about the possible need of surgical drainage later. But, patient insisted him to go for an early drainage, as he wanted to get rid of his sufferings as early as possible. Doctor tried to convince him in different ways, but nothing worked. Finally, as the patient was a farmer, surgeon explained him as—"Early drainage of this swelling will be like early harvesting of your crop. You will waste the manpower and will not get anything out of it." This analogy worked and patient was convinced to continue the conservative treatment.

> After few days on the first consultation, a female patient revisited to her doctor as she was not satisfied with the prescribed treatment. She had been given some medicines whose onset of action was late, but the effect was sustained for a prolonged time. This was explained to her during the first consultation, but somehow, she had missed to understand. She insisted the doctor to change her medicines. But, it was too early to expect any effect from them. So, the doctor explained him with the analogy of oil and water.
>
> *"What happens when you heat oil and water in your kitchen? The water starts boiling in a very short time, but once you stop heating, it cools down early. On the other end, oil takes some time to get hot, but once heated; it remains hot for a longer time. Right? So, the action of this medicine is like heating the oil, and not the water."*
>
> This method worked. She was satisfied by this explanation and agreed to continue with the same medicines.

With increasing experience, a doctor learns more such simple and interesting analogies which can be appropriately used for some difficult situations.

- *Share the source of relevant information:* In today's era, it is becoming a common habit of the patient to search about their disease on internet, before or after consulting a doctor. Many a times, they only land up in a state of panic and confusion. So, it will be better that if possible, doctor should himself share the link of authentic and reliable information about the disease with his patient (e.g., a link of video on proper self examination of breast). In some cases, this method may save his precious time also, as it may not be possible for the doctor to teach him everything in a single visit. Similarly, doctor can also provide some printed information material (e.g., dietary advice, exercises, etc.) from his clinic to the patient.

- *Before and after investigations:* Investigations are only supplementary to a proper clinical diagnosis. But, during present era, there role cannot be ignored in patient's management. Using his knowledge and experience, doctor makes a provisional diagnosis on the basis of signs and symptoms of the patient. Then, he selects some suitable investigation (hematological, biochemical, radiological, etc.) to confirm the diagnosis. It is essential because a wrong diagnosis will lead to a wrong treatment, which will be ineffective or even hazardous also. The result of investigations may confirm or reject the provisional diagnosis.

It is essential to keep explaining the patient about the need, role, and results of various investigations. Following points should be remembered during consultation with the patient:

- Select only the suitable and essential investigations. There is no advantage in advising a battery of investigations in all types of disease.
- Explain him briefly about the provisional diagnosis and the need of the investigation to confirm it.
- In selected cases, give him some idea about the approximate cost of the investigation (e.g., CT scan, MRI, etc.)
- In selected cases, briefly explain him the procedure of investigation also (e.g., FNAC, IVP, etc.). This will reduce his curiosity and anxiety.
- If the patient is quite curious, show him the film of some other patient, if available (e.g., IVP, MRI, etc.).
- Sometimes, on being advised some investigation, patient may show you some old report of the same investigation (e.g., few months old X-ray chest or X-ray spine etc.). Explain him calmly about the possibility of anatomical and physiological changes with time.
- On arrival of the report, explain him briefly about the findings. Tell him that how did it help you in planning his management.
- Sometimes, a normal report is a bad news for some patients, as they feel like it was only wastage of money on some useless test. Clarify their misconception by explain that how even a normal report has helped you in planning the line of his management.
- Some patients may get horrified by some incidental finding in investigation report. Even if they do not ask you, clarify their doubt about it. Some findings are insignificant, but they may be terrifying for the lay persons. For example, pus cells in urine, detection of few enlarged mesenteric lymph nodes in abdominal ultrasonography, etc.

> A patient visited to a doctor with complaints of mild abdominal pain and low grade fever since last few days. After his clinical examination, doctor started the empirical treatment and advised him the some investigations such as CBC, urine test, etc.

Chapter 22: Explanation Skills

> Next day, he collected the investigation reports from the laboratory. He was horrified to find the he was having *2-4 pus cells/HPF* in his urine. Also, some of his reports like *MCV* and *MCHC* were not in the normal range. His anxiety was relieved only when the doctor explained him properly about the significance of these abnormal reports.

- After getting the results of first set of investigations, sometimes some other investigation may be required. For example, advising CT scan to a patient whose ultrasonography has detected a lump in his abdomen. Patient may not be prepared for it, and sometimes may even get annoyed on advising some new investigation. So, he should be again explained properly about the significance of the next line of investigation.
- Not all diseases need some test for confirmation. If patient is curious to know that why he has not been advised any investigation, explain him calmly about it.

- *Explain the line of management:* In many cases, doctor may have to change the line of management of the patient, depending upon the response of the patient, investigation reports, etc. So, in such cases, he should properly inform the patient that he is beginning the treatment with a basic regimen only. If it works, he will prefer to continue with it. But, if it fails to bring the desired effect, he has got *something else* in his mind. This explanation will definitely make the patient come back to him only, if he does not get significant relief from the first regimen (otherwise, he may switch over to some other doctor).

The same rule holds good while advising some investigations to the patient. He should be informed that though hundreds of investigations are available for this disease, but still you would prefer to move step-by-step, keeping patient's comfort and expenditure in your mind. He may need some more investigations in future, depending upon the results of presently advised investigations.

Never underestimate the importance of even trivial knowledge given to your patient. It can sometimes lead to the miraculous positive effects. For example, it is better to explain the patient about the *role and effects* of prescribed medicines. This knowledge may psychology enhance their effect on his body. For example:

> A surgeon stitched some accidental wounds of an old man in minor OT. Then, he prescribed him some medicines and explained him and his relatives about the role of each drug in a simple language. *"This medicine will avoid the risk of any infection (antibiotics), this one will decrease your pain (analgesic), and this one is for your general strength, which will help in early healing of your wounds (multivitamin)."* This simple explanation gave the old man a feeling of psychological satisfaction and well being during healing period of his wounds.

- *Assess the understanding:* For almost all the times, the information about the disease and its management is totally new for the patient. Even if the doctor tells him about it properly, he may or may not understand it, either fully or at least some part of it. Some studies reveal that up to 80% of received medical information is forgotten by the patients immediately and nearly half of the retained information is incorrect.

  So, it is essential for the doctor to keep checking simultaneously about the understanding of the patient. Body language of the patient plays an important role here, most importantly his gesture (head nodding) and facial expressions. If these positive signs are lacking, doctor may have to repeat the information in some different way.

  At the end, the doctor should confirm about the understanding of the patient. In some cases, it is better to ask the patient to tell the doctor about what has been told to him. (This is known as "teach back" method.) This is commonly practiced when patient has been advised to practice something at his home, e.g., How to take the medicines? How to use the inhaler? etc.

  In case of pediatric or elderly patients, it should be confirmed that the person who is taking care of the patient has understood about the management properly.

CHAPTER 23

Persuasion Skills

There are only two sorts of doctors: those who practice with their brains, and those who practice with their tongues.
—*Sir William Osler*

Medical science is a vast and complex field which encompasses the knowledge of various types of diseases and their treatment. A physician acquires this knowledge after many years of studies and it gets augmented with his experiences in clinical practice. On the other hand, a patient is totally inexperienced about the disease and knows almost nothing about human anatomy or physiology.

The most challenging task for a physician is to convince his patient about the seriousness of any disease and the plan of its management. It is essential for him to acquire special skills of persuasion to convince any patient or his family members to accept some major interventions, such as hospitalization, investigation, surgery, etc.

Why is it Difficult?

First of all, it is essential for a doctor to know that why is it a difficult task. The basic instinct of any patient is to get rid of his sufferings in the easiest possible way and that is why, he instinctively avoids any major intervention (such as hospitalization, surgery, etc.) during the course of his treatment.

Let us understand it by imagining a case of some middle-aged man who is suffering from a reducible inguinal hernia since 6 months and has been advised by a surgeon for its surgical treatment. Following are some of the possible reasons which can stop him from accepting the advised surgical treatment:
- *No troubles:* For a person who is carrying an absolutely painless swelling (inguinal hernia) in the most concealed part of his body, surgery will sound like a supra-major kind of treatment. In contrast, a person suffering from severe pain of acute appendicitis

or another person having a swelling on his forehead region is more likely to give the consent for his surgery.
- *Fear of complications:* No doubt that any kind of surgery or anesthesia carries some major or minor complications with it, but presumption of a layperson about the possible complications is much higher than the reality. People are usually very much afraid of any mishappening during or after any kind of surgery or general anesthesia. Bad experiences of some other known person in past adds a major fuel to this fire.
- *Financial expenditures:* In most of the cases, the cost of any hospitalization, major investigation, or surgery is to be paid by patient or his family. So, if he is not under coverage of any kind of insurance scheme, he will have to think about the expenditures, especially if they are beyond his affordability.
- *Disturbance of routine life:* This is probably the most common problem which comes in mind of almost every patient whenever he has to take a decision about his hospitalization or surgery. Any such intervention is definitely going to disturb the regular working schedule of patient and his family, even if he is ready to afford all the expenditures.
- *Is it really needed?* This is another common reason which strikes in patient's mind whenever any major step like hospitalization or surgery is offered to him. Many people have got a habit of confirming any doctor's advice by taking a second opinion from someone else. Some patients may think that probably this intervention is not at all required for their disease and the doctor is offering it to them only for his own benefit. This doubt is more likely to occur if the doctor is not looking confident while informing the patient about his management plan.

HAZARDS OF POOR PERSUASION SKILLS

The news of having any kind of disease is obviously bad for any patient and his family. Moreover, if the disease requires some major intervention (such as hospitalization or surgery) for its treatment, then it becomes even worse for them. Communication of doctor with patient and his family is the most crucial at this point. A half-heartedly conveyed information about the need of some major procedure will further worsen the situation. If the doctor fails to show proper confidence while communicating with them, then it may lead to any

of the following outcomes, which may be hazardous for patient as well as the doctor:
- Patient may get frightened of the advised treatment and may start seeking for some alternative remedies. In some cases, it may only worsen his disease.

> A middle-aged female was found to be having a 15-mm stone in pelvis of her right kidney. A surgeon casually informed her about the need of surgical removal of the stone, without explaining the details properly. She got horrified and started taking some alternative medicines for dissolving the stone, along with the analgesics for her pain, as and when required. After few months, she was brought back to the hospital by her relatives with high-grade fever and vomiting. Investigations revealed that her stone had not only increased in size, but more importantly, it had led to the complication of pyonephrosis. Her right kidney was totally nonfunctioning and was converted into a bag of pus. Moreover, she had also developed severe gastritis because of chronic analgesic abuse.

- Patient may seek a second opinion from some another physician or surgeon. Sometimes, the opinion of the second person may be slightly different from the first doctor. In some cases, this may lead patient and his family in a state of great confusion.

> A 5-year-old child was admitted in hospital with abdominal distension and bilious vomiting. His abdominal X-ray showed features of intestinal obstruction. Surgeon planned for his laparotomy and informed his parents about it. They were not convinced and preferred to take their child to some other hospital for a second opinion. After examining the child, the second surgeon preferred to keep him on the conservative management initially. He explained about it properly to the parents and also informed that he may require surgery if there is no improvement on conservative line. Fortunately, his condition improved in next 24 hours and so, the conservative management was continued for another 2–3 days. Child was discharged without any surgical intervention. The parents defamed the first surgeon in their community for performing unnecessary surgeries on his patients.

- In a long run, if the surgeon or physician repeatedly fails to convince his patients, he may go in a stage of frustration and depression, especially during early stage of his clinical practice. For example, a young surgeon finds that he has consulted 35 surgical cases in his clinic during whole month, but only five of them were operated by him during this period. The rest of the patients never returned back after their first consultation. This was certainly because of some lacunae in his communication and he certainly needed some improvement of his persuasion skills.

HOW TO IMPROVE THE PERSUASION SKILLS?

Whatever the reason may be, a doctor has to develop good persuasion skills to convince the patient and his family to heartily accept the recommended treatment for his disease. First of all, he must try to find out that what is making his patient reluctant in accepting the offered treatment. Then, he should try his best to clarify all the doubts of the patient and his family.

Following are some important suggestions which should be kept in mind to improve your persuasion skills:

- *What is the major reason?* The major reason of reluctance of a patient can be any one or more from the above mentioned list. For example, for the same disease and line of management, one patient may be afraid of the surgical complications and someone else may be worried about the cost. During his communication, the doctor should try to find the real reason which is troubling his patient. It will help him in focusing upon its possible solution in his counseling.
- *Assurance:* If the patient is mainly afraid of the *complications* of surgery or anesthesia, assure him that with the advancement of medical science and technology, surgeries have become safer now. Assure him that the possibility of complications is less than what is being suspected by the patient or his family.
- *Fear kills the fear:* A patient is more likely to accept the offered treatment if he gets convinced that the complications of the treatment are much less than the possible complications of his disease itself.

  Every disease carries the risk of some major or minor complications with itself. During counseling of the patient, doctor should make a habit of informing him properly about the possibility of at least one or two major complications, in a way which is clearly understood by the patient. He should be clearly informed about the risk of treatment versus risk of no treatment for his disease. This should be done as a part of routine counseling, even if the patient does not ask about the possible complications of his disease. This will certainly change his views about the need of advised treatment.

> An elderly person was having inguinal hernia since many years. He had consulted several surgeons during this period and all of them had advised him for surgery. He was hesitant in accepting this line of treatment as his hernia was painless and he was absolutely comfortable otherwise. One surgeon explained him about the possibility of obstruction and strangulation in inguinal hernia, with the help of some diagrams. This was some new information for the patient. Anticipating the fear of this complication, he immediately agreed for his surgery.

- *Real-life incidents:* Examples of some patients, who had similar disease and had accepted or refused the advised treatment, will impart a major impact on patient's thinking. There may be some cases from the experience of the treating physician (or of any other physician) in past. For example:

> A patient was highly reluctant in undergoing surgery for his acute appendicitis. He insisted his surgeon to treat him on conservative line only. The surgeon informed him about the possibilities of complications, but that did not change his mind. Finally, he told him about another patient of acute appendicitis who had visited to the hospital few weeks ago and had also given a negative consent for his surgery. The same patient was brought back to the hospital after few days with severe perforation peritonitis due to ruptured appendix. This example was enough to change the thinking of the new patient.

If possible, patient should be allowed to meet and communicate with the patients who have been successfully cured by accepting the prescribed medical or surgical treatment. This should be done only after taking the consent of the cured patients.

> A patient was afraid of undergoing laparoscopic cholecystectomy for his asymptomatic gallstones, mainly because of his fear for surgery and anesthesia. His surgeon advised him to meet another patient in the ward, who had undergone the same

> procedure. The old patient was absolutely comfortable and was ready to be discharged from the hospital. He shared his experiences with the new patient, mainly about his postoperative period. This greatly reduced the fear and suspicion of the patient and he readily agreed for his surgery.

- *Best possible treatment:* The best impact occurs when you inform the patient that you will prefer to get the *same* treatment if you or any member of your family or any VIP person will get the same disease. This deeply assures the patient that he is receiving the best possible treatment for his disease. For example, parents of a child with inguinal hernia were hesitant to agree for his surgery and were seeking for some alternative remedy. The surgeon confidently said to them—"If tomorrow my own child gets a hernia, I would prefer only and only surgical treatment for him". In another case, an elderly person with pulmonary tuberculosis was reluctant to take the medicines for so long period. His physician persuaded him to continue the prescribed regimen by saying—"Even if our President or Prime Minister suffers from tuberculosis, he will have to take the same medicines for the same duration".
- *Photographs:* The pre- and post-treatment photographs of some old patients with the same disease can play an important role in persuading the patient. These photographs convey several important messages to the patient like:
  - He feels that he is not the only one who has suffered from the disease of so much severity.
  - He gets a positive impression about the capability of his doctor by noticing the difference in post-treatment photograph of the same patient, e.g., fine scar mark, disappearance of pigmented patch, etc. He starts imagining the same outcome with his problem also.

> A young girl visited her family physician with a large mole on her shoulder region. She strongly wished to get rid of it, but the same time, was quite afraid of any surgical intervention. The physician referred her to a plastic surgeon, which showed her few pre- and postoperative photograph of some other female with almost same problem. She was highly impressed by the outcome and so, got convinced to get herself operated by the same plastic surgeon.

Chapter 23: Persuasion Skills

This method is more effective in some specialties, such as dermatology, plastic surgery, etc. It is nice for any doctor to have a good collection of photographs of the patients who have been treated by him. But at the same time, following precautions should be kept in the mind while clicking photographs of the patients:

- Inform the patient clearly about your intention behind clicking his photographs. Tell him that you are also glad to find so good results and so, you would like to show it to the other patients with similar problems or to the other doctors of your field (through presentations in conferences, publications, etc.).
- Ideally, proper consent should be obtained from the patient to avoid any dispute in future.
- Do not include face of the patient in your photographs. Face reveals the identity of any person and so, it should not be included unless absolutely required. Even when included, eyes should be covered or blurred by digital pixelization.
- Additional precautions should be made while clicking photographs of private regions, such as breast, genitals, etc.
- Immediately after clicking, photograph should be shown to the patient to make him sure that his face has not been included in the frame.
- Similarly, name and address of any patient should not be displayed along with the photograph.

> A surgeon had successfully operated upon a patient with a huge inguinal hernia. He had clicked several pre and post operative photographs, mainly to show the impressive outcome of his surgery to the other patients in future. But his only mistake was that he had taken full body view in some photos. After few days, he showed these photographs to some other patient with the same problem. The new patient was surprised to see that the photograph was of a well known person from his village, but no one was aware of his hernia or surgery. In a short time, the news spread all around the village, and the old patient became furious on the surgeon for breaking the confidentiality of his problem.

HOW TO CONVINCE TO AVOID?

This is not the rule that the patients always avoid the major interventions or procedures. On the contrary, in some cases, they insist

the doctor for some intervention which is not at all indicated for their disease. Following are some common examples:
- A patient, who had suffered from minor head injury few days ago, presented to a surgeon in fully conscious state and insisted him for his hospitalization.
- Parents of a 6-month-old child with an umbilical hernia insisted the pediatric surgeon for its surgical correction.
- A female with 6 mm stone in her renal pelvis asked the urosurgeon to remove it surgically.
- A young male with mild headache insisted the physician to go for his MRI of brain.

In such situation, doctor needs some special skills and tactics to convince the patient. Following are some important suggestions:
- Keep yourself calm and do not get annoyed on the patient.
- Try to find out that what is making your patient to think so. For example, a patient with mild headache asked for the MRI only because his friend with similar symptom was found to be having a brain tumor. Vague opinion from some relative or friend may be another source. In some cases, this demand may be simply because of a random internet surfing by the patient.
- Explain the patient about the reason for which you cannot proceed with his request. Tell him that you are following the universal protocol and that no doctor in the world will accept that demand. Explain him the possible plan of management and reassure that you are always there to modify the line of treatment, if it does not work.
- Explain him about the possible side effects of any investigation or intervention (other than the financial loss). Tell him that these procedures should not be taken very casually and should be performed only when there is a clear indication to proceed for them.

> A young female patient presented with mild epigastric pain in outpatient department (OPD) of a hospital. All basic investigations were normal. Doctor suspected it as a case of gastritis and so, prescribed her an antacid and advised to review after 3 days. She started insisting for hospitalization. The hospital wards were flooding with the patients. Doctor explained her that her disease did not require any hospitalization, but she was adamant. When he tried to find the reason behind it, he found that she was afraid of aggravation of her pain in

> nighttime. So, he informed her about the possibility of cross-infection from the other patients. He also assured her that if required, she can reach to OPD or casualty of the hospital, at any time in day or night. This convinced her to continue the prescribed treatment at her home.

- In some adamant cases, a simple logic can be given to the patient that by not accepting his demand, doctor is himself losing a financial benefit. But still, he is not willing to go on that line. This will also give the patient a positive impression about the honesty and intention of the doctor.
- These irrational requests are more common if the patient is not having any financial problem or is covered under some medical insurance. Sometimes, merely accepting the patient's demand and breaking the standard protocol of management may bring an unexpectedly adverse effect to reputation of the doctor.

> A patient visited a young surgeon with complaint of mild abdominal pain. After taking his history and examination, he advised him for some basic investigations, which also included the ultrasonography of abdomen. Patient had heard a lot about CT scan and so, he insisted the surgeon to get his CT scan done (instead of the ultrasonography). He also assured him to not to worry about the financial expenses. Instead of explaining him about the difference between ultrasonography and CT scan, the young surgeon accepted patient's demand. All the reports were absolutely normal, including CT scan. He prescribed him some symptomatic treatment and asked to report back after a week, but the patient was lost from the follow-up. In the next few months, patient visited few more doctors of his city, along with his reports and documents. All of them were surprised that why that surgeon had advised CT scan (instead of ultrasonography) straightway. Patient never revealed the secret to anyone that it was him who had demanded for the CT scan. In a very short time, the young surgeon was defamed in his society for prescribing the costly investigations without proper indication.

Any investigation or procedure of choice should be of doctor's choice and not of patient's choice.

CHAPTER 24

Examination Skills

> It is much more important to know what sort of a patient has a disease than what sort of a disease a patient has.
> —*Sir William Osler*

After taking a detailed history of the patient, proper general and local examination is essential to make a provisional diagnosis of some diseases. At the same time, it should be remembered that the procedure of examination of the patient also plays an important role in the quality of doctor-patient communication.

During the examination, doctor performs various acts on his patient with the help of his hands (mainly during palpation) and various instruments, such as stethoscope, torch, hammer, etc. Though the patient is unable to understand that what the doctor is trying to find out, he feels satisfied if the doctor performs the procedure of examination properly and meticulously.

A young male visited to a surgeon with a painless swelling on his umbilicus since few weeks. During examination, surgeon pressed the swelling juts once and instantly made the diagnosis of umbilical hernia. He advised him for ultrasonography and explained the need of surgery for it. Although the surgeon was absolutely correct in making a provisional diagnosis of umbilical hernia, the patient was not satisfied. He visited to some other surgeon. The second surgeon, after performing the relevant general examination of the patient, performed a methodical local examination of that umbilical swelling. First, he inspected it for few seconds and asked the patient to cough. Then, he palpated it for temperature, asked for any tenderness, then reduced the swelling, palpated for the defect, and again asked the patient to cough. After performing all these procedures, he explained him about the need of investigations and surgery for the umbilical hernia. The whole act of examination took only few minutes, but the patient was immensely satisfied with the diagnosis and line of management of the second surgeon.

Sometimes, doctor is able to make a "spot-diagnosis" of some diseases, mainly by virtue of his experience. But, his art of making an instant diagnosis without performing proper examination may not impress all of his patients. It is true that because of the high patient load, it may not be possible for the doctor to perform a complete and methodical examination of all systems of all patients in his OPD or casualty. But still, he should spend at least few more minutes in performing the relevant examination of the patient. That will not only confirm his spot-diagnosis, but more importantly, will make the patient feel that he is in the hands of a reliable and experienced doctor.

ROLE OF CHAPERON

The privacy and comfort of the patient should be on the top priority during his or her examination. Doctor should not miss any important finding, but at the same time, patient should not feel uncomfortable or embarrassed during clinical examination.

Only required and desired persons should be allowed to be present during examination of patient. Privacy should be maintained by isolating the examination couch with the help of curtain or screen. If there is any CCTV camera in the room, examination couch should never come within the recording area.

Privacy and comfort of patient depend on several factors, such as body part to be examined, age, gender, dressings, culture, religion, etc. Broadly, various body parts of any patient can be divided in three different categories:
1. Exposed parts—e.g., face, palm, back of hand, etc.
2. Exposable in public—e.g., neck, forearm, etc.
3. Exposable in privacy only—e.g., breast, genitals, etc.

There can be some variations in categorization from patient to patient. For example, an elderly lady may comfortably show some lesion on her abdomen to the doctor, but the same cannot be expected from a young female. Doctor should consider all these fact during selecting the most appropriate place for his patient's examination.

As a rule, a female attendant should always be present during examination of a female patient by a male doctor, especially when it is being done in isolation for some body parts such as breast, abdomen, genitals, etc. A female nurse is the ideal person for this job in hospital. She should first prepare the female patient for examination by proper position, covering, etc. She should remain present and visible to the patient throughout the examination. If nurse is not available, some other suitable person, such as female servant should be present during examination of a female patient by any male doctor.

Some female patients feel more comfortable if their examination is conducted in presence of any of their relatives such as mother, sister, husband, etc. This choice should be left to the patient only. If a female nurse is available, there should not be any compulsion of presence of some relative with the patient. For example, a female may like her sister to be present during her abdominal examination by a male doctor. But, she may not like her presence during her genital or rectal examination. This can be decided by some verbal communication and consent before examination. Out of all the available options, husband is usually the best accompanying relative in most of the cases.

Although there is no similar rule for examination of a male patient by a female doctor, still many female doctors prefer to keep a male attendant during isolated examination of any male patient.

AVOID SCANNING DOCUMENTS BEFORE EXAMINATION

Many patients present their old documents (such as old prescriptions, investigation reports, etc.) to the doctor in the very beginning of consultation. Some even insist the doctor to check their old reports before taking any history or performing any examination. Avoid doing so, as it may bias you in some cases. Gently assure the patient that you would go through his file, but only after taking his history and examination.

> A patient presented to a young surgeon's clinic with complaint of abdominal pain since few weeks. Before palpating his abdomen, the surgeon scanned his old investigation reports. It included the report of abdominal sonography which was performed recently by a senior and renowned radiologist of his city. Since the report was normal, surgeon did not pay much attention on dedicated palpation of patient's abdomen. He was having a small *lump* in his epigastric region, which was missed by the radiologist as well as by the surgeon.

Index

Page numbers followed by *f* refer to figure

A
Adapters 49
Addiction 112
Age 63
Alcohol 115
Allergy history 133
Analogies, Use of 210
Anamnesis 14
Answering skills 195
Antenatal history 139
Appetite 107

B
Barriers of communication 35
Birth history 141
Bladder and bowel habits 116

C
Channels of communication 33
Chaperon, Role of 225
Chronological order 79
Clinical diagnosis 16
Closed posture 45*f*, 207*f*
Closed questions 91, 188
Comprehensive history taking 14
Contact history 121
Conversational gestures 48, 206

D
Decoding 28
Developmental history 143
Diabetes, History of 97
Diet 109
Differential diagnosis 15

Distance 53
Drug history 129

E
Encoding 28
Examination skills 224
Explanation skills 201
External distracters 179
Eye aversion 52*f*, 209
Eye contact 51, 177

F
Facial expressions 50, 178
Family history 119
Final diagnosis 17
First degree relatives 119
Formal communication 32
Format of history 61

G
Gestures 46

H
Head nodding 50, 178
Heteroanamnesis 14
Hindu calendar 78
Hospitalization, History of 100
Hypertension, History of 99

I
Immunization history 146
Informal communication 32
Interaction model 32
Internal distracter 179

Intimate zone 53
Iterative hypothesis testing 14

L

Last menstrual period 123
Leading questions 91, 190
Listening skills 177

M

Marital status 118
Mass communication 33
Menstrual history 122

N

Name 63
Negative history 85
Neonatal history 142
Nonverbal communication 42, 161, 206

O

Obstetric history 127
Occupation 67
Onset of disease 81
Open posture 45*f*, 206
Open-ended questions 90, 188
Order of severity 80

P

Paraverbal communication 41, 206
Past history 95
Pediatric history 135
Personal appearance 42
Personal history 105
Personal zone 53
Persuasion skills 215
Photographs 220
Posture 43
Presenting complaints 70
Provisional diagnosis 17

Public communication 33
Public zone 53*f*

Q

Questioning skills 183

R

Receiver 28
Religion 66
Residence 65
Right of confidentiality 202
Rule of Ten 125

S

Second degree relatives 120
Sender 28
Sex 65
Signs 15
Sleep 106
Smoking 114
Social zone 53*f*
Socioeconomic status 69
Sprinter's position 44*f*, 177
Symbolic gestures 47
Symptoms 14

T

Third degree relatives 120
Tobacco chewing 115
Touching 54
Transactional model 31
Transmission model 31
Treatment history 84
Tuberculosis, History of 96

V

Verbal communication 39, 205
Vocal cues 178

W

Weight change 110

EU GSPR Authorised Reprsentative
Logos Europe, 9 rue Nicolas Poussin
1700, La Rochelle, France
Phone: +33 (0) 6 67 93 73 78
E-mail: contact@logoseurope.eu

www.ingramcontent.com/pod-product-compliance
Ingram Content Group UK Ltd.
Pitfield, Milton Keynes, MK11 3LW, UK
UKHW021832140426
5217IPUK00021B/1397